QUESTIONS YOU SHOULD BE ABLE TO ANSWER FOR YOUR OWN GOOD HEALTH:

- How essential is exercise to total health?
- How fit am I?
- How can I determine my ideal body weight?
- What kind of exercise and how much should I do?
- How does exercise relate scientifically to weight control?
- What exercises are good for my heart—and what ones can be dangerous?
- What are the implications of "warm-up," "peak work," and cool-down"?
- Will exercise defeminize the female body?

You'll find out the answers to these questions and lots more when you read "The Official YMCA Physical Fitness Handbook."

The Official
YMCA
Physical Fitness
Handbook

by Clayton R. Myers
Director, YMCA National
Cardiovascular Health Program
National Council YMCA's

Artist: Nick Cardy

POPULAR LIBRARY • NEW YORK

Preface

In 1973, *THE Y's WAY TO PHYSICAL FITNESS* was published. This book, representing the collective efforts of fifty leaders in the field of exercise physiology, sports medicine and physical fitness, was written to help Y Physical Directors administer a simple, yet sophisticated fitness program. A great deal of thanks must be given to all the contributors of this guidebook for their unselfish efforts.

THE OFFICIAL YMCA PHYSICAL FITNESS HANDBOOK has been written to give to the layman valuable information on the subject of getting into and staying in shape. Mr. Clayton R. Myers, with his vast experience in YMCA Physical Education, not only explains completely the steps involved in becoming physically fit (and the reasons behind these steps), but he also covers additional, related areas of importance—such as nutrition. *THE OFFICIAL YMCA PHYSICAL FITNESS HANDBOOK* is a welcome addition to the National YMCA Physical Fitness Program.

Lawrence A. Golding, Ph.D.
Kent State University, 1974

Acknowledgment

*To William Laas, in sincere appreciation
of his major editorial contribution
to the writing of this book.*

Contents

Chapter 1

EXERCISE AND HEALTH

Sent into orbit to study man's ultimate habitat, our solar system and the universe, the Skylab space missions of 1973–74 stumbled upon a major discovery about man's immediate habitat—our own bodies. Almost by inadvertence, Skylab I and II furnished a rare scientific proof that regular exercise is essential to human health.

For many years medical science has proclaimed exercise, along with correct diet, as one of the twin mainstays of physical fitness—but scientific proofs have been somewhat fuzzy around the edges. Usually they lacked what experimenters and researchers call a control. "Exercise is good for you," but exactly how? To what extent? At what penalty if lacking? Without a control, without statistical comparisons to nail down the answers, the value of exercise to health would remain little more than a doctors' hunch. Skylab provided the control.

To set up a control in scientific investigation, the researcher divides an experiment into parallel halves. In testing a new pharmaceutical drug, one group of patients might take the medicine while another, equivalent group are given placebos only. This second group is the control. If only the treated patients get well, one may then logically infer that the new drug made the difference. The untreated control group eliminates the possibility of coincidence.

Such a procedure sounds a bit cold-blooded, which explains why precisely controlled health experiments with human beings are hard to come by. The Hippocratic Oath tugs at a doctor's conscience if, for the sake of science, he should deny a cure to the sick or place a normal person's health in jeopardy. People don't sit still for manipulation like guinea pigs or live out a lifetime in a day like fruit flies.

1

Skylab solved these research problems in two ways: (1) the space missions placed exactly comparable groups of men into exactly comparable situations; (2) the effects on health were compressed into (and could be observed in) a few months.

Weightless in Space

"Skylab" is a nickname for a tube-shaped laboratory vehicle 114 feet long and weighing 85 tons, cruising in orbit about 250 miles from earth. It accommodates three-man crews ferried from Cape Canaveral via an Apollo spacecraft.

Although huge by the standards of space travel, the Skylab is no Astrodome. During missions the crews were cramped for living room and largely restricted to a sedentary work routine. The orbiting sojourn also subjected them for days and weeks to the phenomenon of weightlessness—a factor accentuating the physiological effects of muscular inactivity.

As every TV space-watcher knows, with the pull of gravity eliminated, objects don't drop, they float. An astronaut can walk upside down on the ceiling, but he needs suction cups on his boots to maintain contact with the floor. Inside his body, weightlessness turns vital life processes topsy-turvy.

Muscles that are ordinarily in tension to hold the body upright on earth relax their tension in weightless space. The unburdened spinal column stretches and body fluids rearrange themselves. Astronauts actually grow an inch or two taller and become leaner at the waistline.

The heart has less work to do in pumping blood from the lower extremities because a weightless fluid runs uphill as readily as downhill. Circulation becomes sluggish and distorted. The blood may pool in awkward places and mysterious changes may occur in its chemical composition and cell count.

From the point of view of physical fitness, a weightless sojourn resembles in exaggerated form the situation of a hospital patient lying in bed for many days. When he finally gets up, he has trouble staying on his feet. The same thing happens to astronauts when they return to earth.

This problem of weightless human bodies, serious enough to scare space physicians in the early days of orbital exploration, has relevance to everyday life here on earth. It gives us a concentrated example of the effects of a sedentary life—a lifetime in miniature—of what happens to the human body with no muscular activity or practically none to keep its juices flowing.

On Skylab I

After twenty-eight days in orbit, the three men who lived and worked at sedentary tasks on the mission labeled Skylab I splashed down in the Pacific Ocean. They were understandably wobbly. Such was expected, but the extreme degree of their weakness and disorientation was not expected.

As the astronauts set foot on the recovery ship, the strain of resisting gravity almost knocked them down. They tottered and might have fallen without support. They felt faint and dizzy, off balance, heavy in the lower limbs.

When the astronauts were given various tests of body condition, the test physicians looked grave. The numbers were not good, as doctors say: heart rate, blood pressure, red cell count. All the numbers indicated that three healthy men in the prime of life had suffered an extreme physical deterioration in less than one month.

More alarming still, the weakness persisted. The returned astronauts didn't just walk off and go about their business. For several uneasy weeks, they stumbled around Houston uncertainly, struggling to regain their normal faculties. It was a long pull before test results would show their disused muscles and torpid circulation readapting to life within the pull of gravity and capable of supporting physical exertion.

On Skylab II

The men of the next mission, Skylab II, remained in orbit more than twice as long, a total of fifty-nine days, only a few hours short of two months. Yet when they splashed down, they experienced only a faint echo of the homecoming travail of their predecessors.

The expected feeling of heaviness in the limbs and of lightheadedness began to disappear within a few hours. Within a week, two of the astronauts were cheerfully jogging a mile.

What made the difference? Alarmed by the near-crippling of the first crew, NASA made a basic adjustment in the work routine of the second crew. They equipped the orbiting vehicle with a stationary bicycle, or ergometer. In Skylab II, each man pedaled energetically on the exercise machine for a specified time each day. By this means the space doctors hoped to counter the effects of physical inactivity and weightlessness. The stratagem was spectacularly successful.

The Skylab II crew settled into a groove of work, exercise, food, and sleep so comfortably that the mission commander, veteran astronaut Alan L. Bean, felt they could have stayed in weightless orbit indefinitely.

On Skylab III

As if to prove Captain Bean's point, the third mission, Skylab III, zipped past the fifty-ninth day without incident and on into a third month aloft. Its crew exercised even more vigorously than the previous crew, having added a treadmill to the bicycle ergometer. Physical fitness tests involving blood pumping ability, exercise recovery, and a whirling chair revealed something considered remarkable: not only did the men's medical condition become stabilized after a few weeks, but it actually *improved* later in the flight. Thus the exercise more than compensated for the atrophying consequences of weightlessness and inaction; it achieved a "training effect."

When the astronauts returned to earth after eighty-four days in space, a week short of three months, their physical test results were pronounced completely normal.

The Medical Meaning

Dr. Paul Buchanan, a NASA physician, gave the Skylab II men an ergometer test shortly after splashdown. First a workout on the bicycle machine elevated their heart rates and blood pressure; the test measured how long it took these "numbers" to return to normal. Compared to the results of similar workouts by the same men in advance of the space voyage, the loss in body conditioning was only 10 to 20 percent.

Dr. Buchanan described the test data as "a real landmark in medical history." Putting the exercise machines in Skylab II and III (but not in Skylab I) had created a scientifically

4

valid control. Here were three groups of highly trained men in their thirties or early forties, physically on a par, placed in an identical weightless environment doing identical tasks.

Lacking any means of regular exercise, the first Skylab crew returned to earth greatly weakened and perilously close to collapse.

With regular exercise provided, the next crew stayed in orbit twice as long and yet returned with 80 or 90 percent of physical fitness intact in Dr. Buchanan's tests.

The third crew, with the exercise factor intensified, set a record of eighty-four days in space and returned in normal physical shape or even with body condition improved.

There could be no question that exercise and only exercise had preserved the health of the men of Skylab II and Skylab III. Nor could there be any question that *lack* of exercise had dangerously weakened the men of Skylab I.

Those of us who will never come closer to space travel than a television screen can nevertheless profit by the example. The weightless experience of these astronauts created, in a short time, the effects of a sedentary, inactive life on ordinary people over a long time. If man cannot live by bread alone, neither can he thrive without regular physical activity.

Meet Mr. Flab

Our celebrated modern technology, with all its civilized comforts, seems to be creating in everyday life a condition comparable to weightlessness in space. The machine age has left larger and larger numbers of human beings with less and less physical work to do. Today the average adult American doesn't move a muscle if he can avoid it.

Instead of walking, he jumps into a car; instead of climbing stairs, he takes the elevator; instead of playing games, he watches professionals perform on television . . . and so forth. In the world of industry, automatic machines and power tools take arduous physical labor out of farming, forestry, construction, factory assembly, and a host of other occupations, including housework. More than 50 percent of the labor force today follows service or white collar trades that are largely sedentary.

We seem almost to have lost the use of our legs. Even when out for fresh air and exercise, we ride around a golf course on an electric cart. We put a remote control on the TV so that we don't have to get up from our soft, warm chairs to change channels.

It's an easy life, or so it seems, but if muscles could talk, they would bewail the debilitating life we force them to lead. Laziness ultimately destroys the body, literally puts it out of commission. The deterioration in health from inactivity may take a little longer than the twenty-eight days of Skylab I—it may take twenty-eight years—but the results are inexorably disastrous. The cardiovascular effects, poor circulation and an impaired heart, are particularly dangerous.

The dismal fact is that as a people, Americans today are physically in sad shape—men and women, young and old, rich and poor. Under a doctor's scrutiny, we begin to look and act "middle aged" *in our early twenties*. About half of the young men called up for the armed forces in the recent draft could not pass the basic physical tests. We suffer from a national epidemic of flab.

Poor Diet, Too

Dr. Joyce Brothers once wrote: "We Americans have been called the most overfed, underexercised people in the world. This really is just a polite way of saying we are a bunch of fat slobs." Let's be more charitable. Let's just say that our bodies become soft, weak, and vulnerable to disease through a general acceptance of physical torpor as a happy condition of life.

Body flabbiness is promoted further by the notoriously ill-chosen American diet. In this immensely productive country, capable of supplying the best food in the world in enormous quantities, a large part of the populace suffers from malnutrition—and often by choice. The statistics of the food industry clearly show that Americans actually prefer to consume fats and sugar and sweet soft drinks, as well as highly processed snack foods heavy in calories, dubious preservatives, and chemical adulterants but light in essential nutrients.

The careless American diet of snacks and sweets creates body fat with the efficiency of a lard factory but poorly nourishes the muscles and vital organs. If to the inadequate food we add abuse of alcohol, tobacco, sleeping pills, and other drugs ingested regularly, the fitness picture grows even

6

worse. Body flab is not just hyperbole, not a joke: it is a national epidemic. And it's time for a change.

How We Got This Way

It's easy to observe the effects of sloth and overfeeding. Every pet owner knows that the best way to kill a healthy pup or kitten is to stuff it with food and keep it inactive. Such famous physicians as the late Dr. Paul Dudley White have scolded us for years on the fatal combination of rich food and inactivity. We may wonder, then, why poor body condition has been so long neglected as a serious public health problem.

Historically, the problem has been sneaking up on us over generations of time. Primitive man survived largely through his physical exertions. He hunted animals and he fought other men. He and his wife labored in the fields or gathered food in the woods and lifted water, almost constantly in physical action. The human body that evolved out of this rugged lifestyle still remains with us in essential outline, but the motivations for physical effort have vanished. Modern man survives largely by his mental efforts, his wits and skills, which he increasingly exercises sitting down. If we could combine man's past vigor and activity with our present medical advances—it would be ideal.

The advance of civilization basically matches the progressive substitution of brain for brawn. The invention of labor-saving methods and machines traditionally has been hailed as a social good and has made its inventors rich men. Today it looks as if we have finally had too much of a good thing. Our cleverness leaves most of us so free of physical stress and movement that today's principal work problem is not hardship or drudgery but sheer boredom.

In all of the current emphasis on ecology and the preservation of natural resources, the wastage of one national resource has been overlooked. Item by item, technology has been eating into the quality of the human body. Physical activities once prevalent in daily life have almost vanished, such as walking to school or work, climbing stairs, carrying coal, water, or food supplies, chopping wood, picking berries, washing clothes. Now we leave as much of that as we can to autos and automation.

7

Why Body Conditioning?

Because of the many laborsaving devices used today (and this is progress), individuals must purposely plan an exercise program. They need to develop awareness that underutilized bodies can threaten good health and possibly mental equilibrium as well. Some would call the decline of physical fitness in so large a part of the population a threat to our survival as a nation.

Mr. or Mrs. or Miss or Ms. Flab is in trouble, and fortunately, is beginning to realize it. That's why we have diet fads and "instant physical culture" such as sauna baths and electric massage. These are symptoms and gropings for a solution. In truth, as in efforts to preserve the natural environment, there is no quick magic to body conditioning or reconditioning. It takes steady application and a new attitude toward preserving the natural values that make life worth living.

The simple fact is that a long-range trend of slow physical decline now menaces our lives like the plagues of other centuries. Heart disease and related circulatory ailments are today the leading cause of death in the United States. Ways must be found to reverse the trend, to restore our bodies to their natural bounce and beauty. Ecology begins at home.

Fortunately the way to better body conditioning and physical fitness is now well understood—a combination of *sound* diet and *regular* exercise. To produce results, the methods used must be scientifically correct and yet within reach of the average person going about his business every day. They must also be enjoyable—fun to do and rewarding in terms of a better life. That is the proposition of this book.

The "Y" Way

The approach to body conditioning described here is not mere theory nor is it faddish extravaganza. It starts with the assumption that fit body condition is important to you and worth making a small effort to achieve.

The methods given in this book have been developed within the world's most experienced physical fitness organization, the Young Men's Christian Association. The YMCA doesn't just talk physical fitness or write books about it; the "Y" movement deals with real, live people of both sexes and of all races and types seeking good health, throughout this country and in many other parts of the world.

The strongest recommendation for the "Y" way to physical fitness is that these methods work. They have worked for 40 million members over the years. They are practical, common sense, scientific, and not at all difficult to follow. The "Y" way of body conditioning can work wonders for you.

Chapter 2

SHAPE UP TO LIVE!

The YMCA has guided millions of persons in the direction of physical fitness and in so doing has developed a safety-proven, common-sense approach to exercise that totally rejects the faddist or cultist approach.

There are many definitions of physical fitness, but the best one is the simplest. To be physically fit is to be in good health. To be unfit is to be in poor health.

Even if no obvious symptoms of illness appear, a person in anything less than good physical condition cannot operate at peak efficiency and cannot enjoy life as it is meant to be enjoyed. On the negative side, such a person also stands in very real danger of disabling disease and sudden death.

Body conditioning is a procedure, a means to the end of attaining physical fitness. For most people the procedure consists of combining proper diet and regular exercise. But it involves something more: a state of mind. A person who seriously undertakes to restore his body adopts a new attitude toward life.

He dedicates himself to health. He rejects unhealth. He becomes suspicious of self-indulgence. If self-discipline is required, he accepts the necessary degree of discipline. He will willingly make the minor sacrifice of lazy comfort or of his sweet tooth for the major benefit of good health. He reminds himself constantly that the greatest benefit of body conditioning for physical fitness may be life itself.

The Sedentary Syndrome

Medically, physical fitness is not just a general term but a specific one: the ability of the body to respond to work or

11

stress. The body's condition—its ability to meet the demands put upon it—may be measured accurately by a series of fairly simple tests. The combined results of these tests establish a fitness score—and the problem today is that in the American population the fitness score has fallen, is falling, and will continue to fall unless the trend is reversed.

Professor Thomas K. Cureton of the Physical Fitness Laboratory, University of Illinois, has said:

"The average American young man has a middle-aged body. He can't run the length of a city block, he can't climb a flight of stairs without getting breathless. In his twenties, he has the capacity that a man is expected to have in his forties.

"The average middle-aged man in this country is close to death. He is only one emotional shock or one sudden exertion away from a serious heart attack—this nation's leading cause of death."

The statistics are pretty chilling, all right. Coronary heart disease, the classic "heart attack," today accounts for about four out of every ten deaths from *all* causes (including accidents, suicide, and congenital malformations, which are not diseases). This is more than the combined total of deaths from cancer, flu, pneumonia, diabetes, and ulcers. When other ailments involving blood circulation are added—stroke, arteriosclerosis, hypertension—*every second death in the United States* is cardiovascular in origin.

America has the grim distinction of leading the world in deaths per capita from cardiovascular deficiencies, about one million persons a year in round numbers and about half of the men who die between 45 and 65. Even more alarming is the gradual but persistent spread of what formerly was a syndrome of the middle-aged male to more and more women, more and more young people, and even to children. Our life expectancy, which had been rising steadily since the 19th century, has now turned downward. We're not living as long, on the average. Already, about one out of every ten deaths, male and female, before age 35 is blamed on heart disease.

The relation of heart and circulatory troubles to physical fitness or unfitness would seem so obvious as to go without saying. Yet until fairly recent years, heart attacks were blamed on sudden exertions or heavy emotional stress, and the victims were instructed to rest. Today we know that while shocks and strains may bring on a coronary, the underlying

12

cause is a state of physical deterioration that may have been in progress for a long time.

Cardiovascular deterioration may be arrested. In younger people it may be reversed. And the principal way of coming to the rescue is exercise.

Elements of Fitness

Although many things contribute to a well-conditioned body, the key to all is the circulation of blood. No part of the body can survive without a constant supply of blood from the heart and lungs. It may survive but cannot thrive if the supply, even though sufficient for bare existence, is insufficient to support activity and growth.

The bloodstream carries nutrients and especially oxygen to every cell of the body, in order to fuel every output of energy from walking and eating to thinking and sex. One of its principal functions is the exchange of oxygen for waste materials in the process of metabolism—and it is this exchange that has been directly related to exercise or the lack of it.

Modern fitness tests include such quantitative measures as oxygen uptake and oxygen consumption (especially the amount of oxygen supplied to the heart in relation to the amount used up by the heart muscle); air exchange in the lungs; the volume of blood pumped by each heart stroke; the heart rate or pulse; and blood pressure in the arteries. The resulting numbers directly or indirectly measure a person's stamina and endurance.

These concepts may seem highly technical or esoteric until one appreciates their application to daily life. Some years ago an experiment in California measured the blood circulation of 500 factory workers. Like most Americans, these people had found little physical activity convenient to them after the age of 22. The measurements showed that the average teenager's circulation had dropped 40 percent by the time he was twenty-five years old. By age thirty, he had lost 60 percent.

The good news is that this process of deterioration, which is closely associated with aging, need not be accepted as inevitable. Obviously, some general wear and tear of the body cannot be avoided over the years. On the average, a 60-year-

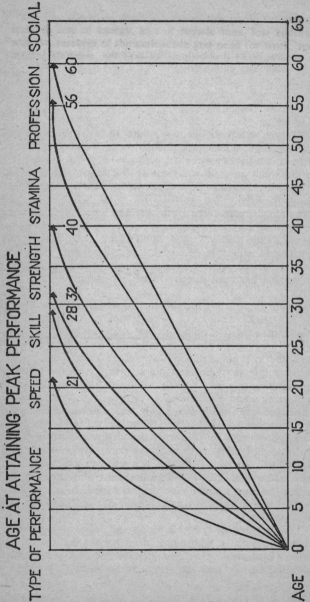

old has about 70 percent of the maximum oxygen uptake of a 25-year-old. But averages are deceiving. Professor Per-Olof Astrand of Sweden, one of the world's outstanding authorities on physical medicine, puts it this way:

"If two 50-year-olds are identical in endowment but one is trained [i.e., systematically exercised] and the other untrained, then the trained person would have an oxygen uptake ability—and maximum motor power—on the same level as the untrained person had around the age of 35 to 40. In other words, moderate training can lead to a ten-to-fifteen-year biological rejuvenation."

Exercise can take ten or fifteen years off your physiologic age! Surely a compelling motive for body conditioning—now!

Penalties of the Unfit Life

Without belaboring the point, it seems clear that the principal cause of physical deterioration derives from subjecting the body to unnatural stresses. The Cardiovascular Disease Risk Profile on page 98 lists a number of factors increasing the probabilities of heart disease that result from bad habits: cigarette smoking, high blood pressure, obesity, elevated levels of cholesterol and triglycerides in the blood (blood fats), lack of physical activity in daily life, and control of stress and tension.

All of these factors are interrelated and their combined effect is more than additive.

The body can adapt itself to inactivity just as it adapts to heat, cold, altitude, or hard labor. Unfortunately, we are

The graph shows the relationship between age and fitness in various pursuits, according to athletic records and other data. Thus at age 21 a man may attain peak physical performance in speed (as a runner), at age 28 in skill (e.g., as a ball player), at age 32 in strength (a weight lifter), and at age 40 in stamina (a jogger or marathon runner). But in non-athletic pursuits he continues rising toward his professional peak as a business executive, doctor, etc., at about age 56, and toward his social peak in the community or in politics at age 60 or beyond. The graph is based upon a concept developed by Alexander Melleby, Physical Education Director, New York City YMCA.

scarcely aware of adapting to *dolce far niente* until we try to put the unused body in action, as in running to catch a bus.

In an extreme case of inactivity, prolonged bed rest, experiments have disclosed strange reactions including decalcified bones, reduced blood volume, shrinking muscle size, impaired heart output, and a marked increase in heart rate. The subjects felt dizzy; some fainted when they first stood on their feet. An exertion which normally raised the heart rate to 120 beats per minute required 170 beats per minute after a few weeks of bed rest. We have already referred to the comparable effects on astronauts in weightless space.

In the reverse direction, physically trained persons reduced the heart rate required for specific work loads and oxygen uptake more than doubled.

Benefits of Activity

In modern life, one has to begin to look upon his body as almost another entity, a partner to the mind, and if you like, a responsibility to God. We take better care of our automobiles than we do of our personal vehicles of flesh and blood. Athletes know full well that they must train; the rest of us should come to the same appreciation of what life is all about. We may not intend to break any records, but we need *extra* physical activity just to counter the fatal consequences of the habitual sedentary life.

Physical activity can make you healthier, happier, *and younger*. A firm body glowing with health can make you more sexually attractive—and active. Approach your body conditioning program in that spirit. Beware of the easy way.

We read an advertisement for a "health secret" that sounds miraculous. It consists of exercises that "can be performed in just a few minutes with absolutely no huffing and puffing . . . without working up a sweat . . . a way to be fit and trim without working for it." Too good to be true? Let your own common sense give the answer.

You *can* regain the sort of physical condition that was a blessing of happy youth, that makes life fully worth living, but it stands to reason that meaningful exercise will take work, hard work. Yes, it will take two or three months of hard work—of huffing and puffing and working up a sweat.

Twenty years ago an exercise class in a big city YMCA

might number half a dozen people, all of them men, phlegmatically and perhaps a bit grimly going through a set series of calisthenic routines. Today the same class under the same instructor might crowd 100 persons on a gymnasium floor, perhaps half of them women, imbued with a combination of determination and verve. The demand for physical fitness training is growing at an unprecedented rate. The reason is plainly the awakening of the American consciousness to a realistic appreciation of what physical fitness involves.

In our civilization the simple fact is that body conditioning —the systematic improvement of the body—has become as essential to health as clean air and good water. Anyone who is in poor shape, at any age from 20 to 65, has reason for serious concern. He or she is on the way to discomfort and premature aging. His or her life may be in danger. He or she may be missing life's dearest rewards.

Body Conditioning Today

Thanks to the work of physiologists in recent decades, the concept of body conditioning has changed radically in the present generation. As an ideal of the physically fit, we no longer envisage a Charles Atlas, with the bulging muscles, or even a 300-pound defensive tackle on the Miami Dolphins. We now know that the real criteria of good body condition are endurance and stamina, grace, agility, muscle tone, flexibility, and balance, rather than brute strength.

Older tests of muscle strength and power now play a minor role in the scientific approach to physical fitness. So do sports such as bowling, golf, or softball which are essentially tests of skill. Today, because of the emphasis on cardiovascular fitness we want to know how efficiently a person can run, swim, jog, or walk. We encourage dancing, mountain climbing, back-packing in the woods. We sensibly attune the work attainment levels to differences in age, sex, and presence or absence of individual health problems.

Good body condition can mean a lot to you in many ways related to health: a prettier or handsomer appearance, with glowing face and bright eyes; a sharper mind; greater ability and endurance at work or at sports. Good health is more than just an exercise program—although exercise is the keystone of the arch. The healthy life includes eating a balanced diet, observing good habits such as avoidance of alcohol, nicotine, and drugs, and periodical attention to health through medical checkups.

We hope this book can help you to develop a philosophy of health that will at the same time make it fun. Body conditioning leads the way in everyone's pursuit of happiness.

How Fit Are You?

The condition of your body can be described in different ways: as fat or lean; as having a strong heart and robust circulation or the opposite; as lively or prone to fatigue; as resistant to disease or susceptible to it; as muscular or weak in strength—and many others. Literally hundreds of tests are used to measure fitness in various areas and functions of the body.

Some of the more sophisticated tests are described later in this book, in some cases with instructions for self-administering. At this point, however, you might like to get a quick idea of your own body condition by a few simple tests that are revealing but need no special preparation or equipment. You need only strip to your underclothes or night clothes and perform them in your own home. The "passing scores" for some of these tests are as proposed by Prof. Thomas K. Cureton in 1965.

1. Body Conformation

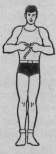

Holding a tape measure, stand with shoulders back and chest expanded with the deepest breath you can

18

hold. Measure the circumference of your chest with the tape just beneath the armpits. Then measure your waist with the stomach relaxed (not sucked in). For a man, the chest should measure five inches more than the waist. For a woman, the difference should be ten inches.

2. Body Balance

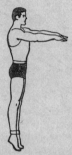

Stand on your toes with heels together and arms extended straight in front of you. Close your eyes. Hold this position for twenty seconds without opening your eyes or shifting your feet.

3. Agility

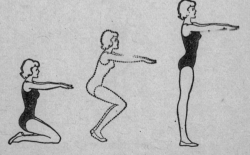

Kneel on the floor with toes extended back and soles of the feet facing up. Stretch your arms forward from the shoulders. Then swing the arms down and up, and jump to a standing position with both feet at the same time, while maintaining your balance.

4. Muscular Power

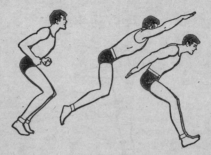

Do a standing broad jump; that is, jump forward as far as you can *without* taking a running start. The length of your jump from this fixed position should approximately equal your height.

5. Endurance

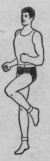

Run in place for one minute, lifting your feet at least four inches from the floor. If this leaves you breathless and with a heart rate over 100, you need training.

6. Flexibility

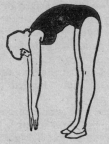

Stand with legs together and knees locked. Men: Bend at the waist and touch floor with fingertips. Women: Bend at the waist and touch floor with palms of hands. *Caution:* If you can't touch the floor as indicated, don't try to force it by "bouncing" downward. This could strain the back. To improve flexibility, you will need a systematic exercise program.

7. Strength

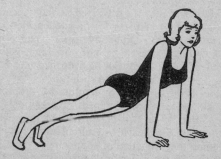

Lie face down on the floor. Place hands on the floor at shoulder level. Fully extend arms to raise the body with back and legs held straight. Lower the body until chest is approximately one inch from the floor. Repeat without bending hips or knees. Men should be able to do eight to ten of these push-ups; women, four to six.

What the Tests Mean

Body conformation is the outward or superficial aspect of body condition. If your waist is much greater around than your chest in expansion, you most likely are overweight. Excess fat gathers around the waistline in a "spare tire" that suggests the presence of excess fat in other parts of the body as well. See Chapter 5 for an accurate method of ascertaining the percent of fat in the body and determining your ideal, or well-conditioned weight.

Body balance comes with good neuromuscular control. The nerves and muscles must work together in actions like dancing, skiing, skating, riding, most ball games, and many of the routine skills of everyday life. Poor performance in balance activities can be improved through practice.

Agility refers to that aspect of motor fitness which enables the body to react quickly. It takes controlled and nimble movements—agility—to spring quickly to one's feet, to hit a baseball or catch a football, to vault a fence, to mount a horse, etc. It is important in body conditioning because an agile person can do more without risking injury, and can control his body quickly and effectively in an emergency. No one should even drive a car, much less play an athletic game, without this physical quality.

Muscular power may be described as the capacity to exert a substantial amount of force with a sudden motion. It is the key element in many competitive sports, since power determines how far a ball can be hit, how far a javelin can be thrown, how high the body can be propelled into a jump or a pole vault, how fast a runner can sprint.

Endurance is the capacity for continued exertion. In cardiovascular training, greater endurance is the key objective. During the first minute or two of activity an oxygen debt may be created, then the heart and circulatory system respond by speeding up their function of supplying oxygen. In popular terms, exertion leaves a person "breathless" until the oxygen supplies are adequate to meet the higher demands. Endurance can be definitely increased by training, even in persons over 60 and, in many cases, even in persons who have suffered a coronary heart attack.

Flexibility means ability to move the joints, the opposite of being stiff or having limited range of movement. It is related to agility in that a flexible body can easily handle a broad range of movements, not limited by pain or "creakiness" in the joints. Exercises that involve bending at the waist, twisting the trunk, pointing the toes, and other such manipulations are aimed at improving flexibility.

Strength has been de-emphasized in the present emphasis in physical fitness, which once advocated the development of rippling, bulging muscles. It is important, however, that certain muscles of the arms, legs, and especially the trunk be strong enough to exert considerable force. Strength exercises in a fitness program today zero in on muscles of the back and chest, essential to climbing; muscles of the buttocks, involved in running, jumping, or cycling; the long back muscles that hold the trunk erect and anchor it against pushing or pulling; and the abdominal and thigh muscles that reinforce the legs in running, jogging, swimming, and many other kicking or leg-lifting actions. Strength figures importantly in hundreds of other everyday tasks, and specific exercises for all major muscle groups should be included in a complete fitness program.

How About You?

These tests merely hint at revealing aspects of physical fitness, but they can help you make an important decision. Let it be stated bluntly: if you "fail" even one of these tests, your exercise program is lacking in some respect and you should secure the counsel of a trained physical educator without delay.

If you can pass all of the tests, you are probably in pretty good condition at this moment. You should consider then whether you are likely to maintain your good physical condition under the circumstances of your daily life.

Don't forget that physical fitness is not a commodity that can be stored. It must be renewed. A continued exercise regimen will help to maintain your body at an efficient level and keep you feeling good, feeling alert, feeling energetic. Appreciate that what you have is precious. Don't let it slip away.

Chapter 3

EAT BETTER TO LIVE BETTER

In youth, the healthy body responds easily and nimbly to any physical demands we make of it. The eyes are sharp, the hearing keen, the brain alert, and so are the muscles. What happens in later life will depend upon habits. Good lifelong habits preserve physical fitness, bad habits dissipate health. The processes are sometimes slow, stealthy, scarcely noticeable, until many years have passed. In adulthood and middle age, the results of health habits make themselves evident for good or ill. Nowhere is this principle more evident than in nutrition.

A healthy existence rests on three foundation stones: adequate rest, nutritious diet, and sufficient exercise. For most Americans, getting enough rest presents few problems. We have trouble getting enough exercise. And we have a great deal of trouble with diet. Every few months, it seems, someone comes along with a sensational "new" diet for losing weight. Only a few work, and most weight loss is only temporary.

Quick-loss diets are boring and unsatisfying so we don't stay with them very long. Some freakish diets leave the body depleted and undernourished. So the dieter abandons each latest miracle, buys another book, and tries something else. What he really needs, instead, is to change the eating patterns, the food *habits*, that are doing him in. With a well-conceived diet and a moderate amount of exercise, no one should ever weigh more than he did in his twenties.

The Logic of Diet

The facts about human nutrition may be briefly stated and are not difficult to understand. Anyone interested in the state of his health should take a little time to study nutrition—to learn the facts and the common sense of food; and studiously disregard the faddists, quacks, mystics, or advertising copywriters and their traps for the unwary, the innocent, or the gullible.

Recent surveys suggest that many Americans, including the affluent as well as the ghetto poor, suffer from malnutrition. Yet other statistics show that two out of every five Americans are obese. How is it that Americans can be both undernourished and overfed at one and the same time?

To a large extent, the answer lies in our eating habits and in food choices made out of heedlessness or ignorance. Only in rare instances does the *quantity* of food became a material diet factor in this country; it is the *kind* of food that makes the difference. Too often the wrong things to eat have a tempting taste or have received the most artful TV advertising commercials.

In the supermarket a woman shopping for food confronts an array of thousands of items that leaves her dazed. Despite some recent progress in labeling food packages with nutritional values, a lot of it is gobbledygook to Mrs. Shopper, and anyway, she has to please her family, watch that food dollar, and save her time. In her train of thought, nutritional needs bring up the rear. The typical homemaker appears to have very limited knowledge of the nutritive values of various foods and only a hazy idea of how to apply such knowledge as she has. Her husband eating a "businessman's lunch" in a snack shop or restaurant doesn't do any better. The logic of a nutritious diet should always be kept in mind. "You are what you eat," says an old adage. You are also a creature of what you fail to eat.

In the nutritional field, what you don't know can hurt you.

Elements of Diet

To many, the definition of health is freedom from disease. Hence if they're not sick, they consider themselves in good health. Children feel good just from the sheer exuberance of

26

being young, so brimming with vital force as to brush aside many a menacing infection or crippling injury. But adults who are not sick are not really in good health either—unless they are physically fit.

In work, at school, in social life, in sports, we perform only as well as our physical well-being allows. Body conditioning is more than a medical antidote for heart disease or a preventive of future agonies. It pays off right now. In relation to diet, a fit person eats well to live better.

There are about fifty known nutrients (and possibly others not yet discovered), which have been chemically classified as proteins, carbohydrates, fats, vitamins, and minerals, plus water. No single food, not even mother's milk, contains all the nutrients we need in the proper amounts we need. In time the infant must be weaned, for the race of man is omnivorous. A good diet for adults must consist of a variety of foods and contain a balance of all important nutrients.

The effects of a diet deficiency or imbalance are slow and subtle but inevitable. People "put on weight" from eating too much or are "always tired" from not eating enough of the right things. A number of diseases, some of them serious, are directly related to diet deficiencies, among them rickets, pellagra, scurvy, beri-beri, goiter, anemia, marasmus, and night blindness.

Captain James Cook accidentally invented nutritional science on a two-year voyage in the eighteenth century when he forced the crew to drink lime juice. Not one sailor died of scurvy, until then the scourge of men at sea. We now know the cause: lack of vitamin C, which Captain Cook supplied in his lime juice. But men continued skeptical and scornful; thus the British sailor acquired a derisive nickname, "Limey."

Nutritionally good food need not cost any more than nutritionally inadequate food, and may often cost less. A common frustration of social workers is the sight of their impoverished clients buying potato chips, candy bars, or frozen cakes costing ten times as much as the raw materials and yet of little nutritional value.

What Nutrition Terms Mean

In this weight-conscious age, everyone knows about calories —that if you take in too many you gain weight. But that is by no means the whole story. A calorie is not something to eat but a measure of food value in one aspect only: energy. It is possible to eat 1,500 calories a day and feel marvelous or to eat 2,000 and feel ill.

Calories

As used in nutrition, one calorie produces enough heat energy to raise the temperature of one kilogram (2.2 pounds) of water one degree Celsius (Centigrade). Technically it is a *large calorie,* abbreviated kcal, and equivalent to 1,000 of the small calories used in your physics and chemistry classes. The body "burns" (oxidizes) food calories to energize our physical activities and stoke the engines of all body processes from thinking to digestion. As in an automobile engine, motive power depends upon efficient use of the fuel.

The number of calories required by the body depends on (1) size, (2) sex, (3) age, and (4) activity. A rough rule of thumb allows 15 kcal per pound of body weight for a maintenance diet, on which one neither gains nor loses weight. However, physical activity does burn up more calories, and older people require less than growing youngsters. Here is a simplified calorie table from information compiled by the National Research Council:

Approximate Daily Calorie Requirements of Normally Active People

Age	Men (154 lbs.)*	Women (128 lbs.)*
25	2,900 kcal	2,100 kcal
45	2,600 kcal	1,900 kcal
65	2,200 kcal	1,600 kcal
	Boys (134 lbs.)	Girls (117 lbs.)
15–18	3,400 kcal	2,300 kcal

*154 lbs. is the average weight of American men of medium build and 5′ 9″ tall; 128 lbs. is the equivalent for women 5′ 4″ tall.

Carbohydrates and fats are the chief food sources of calories, but some may also come from protein foods. One gram (1/30th ounce) of various nutrients supplies the following number of calories:

Carbohydrate	4 kcal
Protein	4 kcal
Fat	9 kcal

It is evident that fat is a concentrated source of calories, providing more than twice as much energy by weight as an equal amount of either carbohydrate or protein. One can readily understand why reduced intake of rich gravies, spreads, cream dressings, etc., is advised for those who are overweight. It is also plain that since *all* categories of nutrients furnish calories, so must the *total* food intake be decreased in a successful reducing diet. Alcohol is a "sleeper" source of calories, often not taken into account by dieters.

Proteins

The word *protein* is derived from the Greek meaning "primary, holding first place." Proteins are indeed the No. 1 consideration in composing any diet. Their complex structure holds the answer to the unsolved riddle, "What is life?" A protein contains nitrogen and sometimes sulphur in addition to carbon, hydrogen, and oxygen, formed into more than twenty different amino acids, which are linked into a chain-like molecular structure. An almost unlimited number of different proteins are possible in the various patterns and combinations of amino acids.

The body can manufacture some amino acids, but not all. The latter must be supplied by foods we eat every day and are known as *essential amino acids*. The nutritional value of a protein depends on the number and kind of amino acids it contains, especially the essential ones. These are broken down by the body and reconstituted to make body proteins.

Proteins are essential building blocks for the growth, maintenance, and replacement of body tissues. They are parts of the structure of skin, hair, nails, connective tissue, and innumerable other organs. Hormones and enzymes are proteins or protein derivatives. A protein deficiency in the diet can be a serious matter. A disease called kwashiorkor kills young children in Asia, Africa, and other parts of the world where the diet consists almost exclusively of starches without proteins.

Lean meat, fish, dairy products, nuts, peas, beans, and whole grains are good sources of protein. However, some of the vegetable sources are not of as good quality for human consumption as the animal sources because they do not contain all the essential amino acids.

The preciousness of good proteins is reflected in traditional cookery. Thus Italian spaghetti sauces, Mexican chili con carne, Indian curries, and our own sandwiches and dumplings were created centuries ago to stretch scarce supplies of animal protein by adding to it cheaper starchy foods.

Proteins cannot be stored in the body to any great extent, hence cannot safely be omitted from a diet aimed at reducing weight. Not only the right amounts but the right kinds of amino acids must be present if the body is to put together the hosts of specific molecules it requires.

Carbohydrates

Carbohydrates similarly are broken down and rebuilt in the body. They are molecules formed of carbon, hydrogen, and oxygen by green plants and utilized in the body in the form of glucose, galactose, and fructose. They include sugars, starches, and cellulose which, together with fats, are the primary sources of fuel for physical processes and activity. The body produces energy by oxidizing these molecules into carbon dioxide and water.

The body can synthesize carbohydrates from other materials, but only in the presence of certain so-called nonessential nutrients. That is why a *variety* of foods must be eaten to power the metabolic machine.

Modern foods rich in carbohydrates include mainly bread, cereals, rice, macaroni, and other grain products; sugar and sweets of any kind; and various root vegetables such as potatoes and beets. The body can transform carbohydrates into portions of the protein building blocks or into fat, which it may store if supply exceeds daily needs.

Fats

A fat is another compound of carbon, hydrogen, and oxygen, but in the form of fatty acids and glycerol, known as glycerides or lipids. Certain fatty acids cannot be synthesized by the body and must be supplied by the diet. They are a major energy source, also essential in digestion, but often overdone in the American cuisine. Nutritionists consider a fat content in the diet of 25 to 33 percent a good diet balance, but 40 percent fat is more typical in practice.

A fat is called saturated when all possible hydrogen bonds in its molecular structure are filled. Otherwise it is unsaturated. Generally, saturated fats are solid at room temperature, while unsaturated fats are liquid (coconut oil, a saturated fat, is an exception).

A monounsaturated fat (olive oil, chicken fat, peanut oil) has one carbon atom free of hydrogen. A polyunsaturated fat (corn oil, soybean oil, fish oils, etc.) has two or more free carbon atoms. Some of the fatty acids (but not all) are essential in the body, which breaks them down and reconstitutes them into fats characteristic of the various tissues.

The saturated fats, mostly from the animal kingdom (bacon, butter, marbled steak, eggs) are suspected of promoting the excess of cholesterol in the blood and thereby the risk of cardiovascular disease.

Cholesterol is a natural, fatty substance manufactured in the human body by the liver. It plays an important role in many physiological processes, digestive juices, sexual secretions, and the brain. However, excess amounts of cholesterol in the blood serum have been associated with atherosclerosis, in which the arteries become narrowed and obstructed by lipids, or fatty deposits.

Since cholesterol is plentiful in foods containing animal fats, early researchers concluded that a chain linkage existed between eating saturated fats in the diet and increased symptoms of atherosclerosis. Some authorities now consider this too simple an explanation, since if we didn't eat cholesterol the body would manufacture it from foods such as potatoes and string beans. Children sometimes appear to inherit a high cholesterol level. In laboratory tests, actually, cholesterol came into prominence as an index of blood-fat levels principally because it was easy to measure. Some nutritionists now shift their emphasis to another indicator of fat in the blood, the serum triglycerides.

The complete truth of the cholesterol matter could take decades to pin down. Certainly too much has been made of it for commercial exploitation. An ad for a margarine proclaims, "Rich in polyunsaturates, too!" implying that the more you eat, the better for you. The authorities agree only on a "prudent diet" with a reduced intake of fats—whether saturated or unsaturated—to reduce the risk of cardiovascular disease as well as obesity.

Vitamins

The vitamins are special chemicals needed in very small amounts to enable the body to perform its complex chemical reactions. They cannot be synthesized by the body, and are not nutrients in the sense of supplying energy or building tissue. They serve as catalysts that speed up the main physiological engine and make it run smoothly. A vitamin deficiency can lead to body deterioration or disease, but such a pathological deficiency is quite rare if one eats a balanced diet.

Some vitamins are lost in food processing (e.g., milling flour, making "instant" potatoes, pasteurizing milk). Where important to health these deficiencies have been tracked down and partly corrected by law. "Enriched" bread, cereals, and milk have had some of the lost vitamins artificially restored. So far as known at present, there is no difference between vitamins derived from natural sources and those synthesized in the chemist's vat. One should remember that all foods are "chemicals" and that even the simplest cookery is a "chemical process."

Whether supplementary vitamins should be added to the diet poses a complex and controversial question. Extra vitamins are no doubt desirable at certain periods, as in pregnancy and early infancy, and in prolonged illnesses associated with loss of appetite or digestive function and poor eating habits. But large doses of some vitamins, particularly A and D, can be toxic.

Not long ago, the New York *Times* reported, a food faddist in England drank a gallon a day of carrot juice, rich in carotene, which the body converts into Vitamin A. His complexion turned a bright orange yellow, and he died of cirrhosis of the liver.

The rationale of taking vitamin supplements is the fear that many people for various reasons find it difficult to obtain and eat a normal balanced diet containing all the essential vitamins. It's easier for them to pop pills and "play safe."

Since unneeded vitamins of most (though not all) types are simply and harmlessly excreted by the body, nothing's lost but the cost. Here again, the passage of time may prove the therapeutic value of vitamin supplements to a normal person's diet, but as of now, most medical opinion considers them largely unnecessary and, in some cases, risky.

The vitamin content of foods and food supplements often is given as a percentage of Minimum Daily Requirement (MDR). The MDR standards are established by the Food and Drug Administration for product labeling to inform the consumer. They are not to be confused with the Recommended Dietary Allowance (RDA) published by the National Research Council. Generally the RDA is greater than the MDA, as in the following table:

	MDR (Adults)	RDA (Man aged 25)
Vitamin A,		
USP units	4,000	5,000
Thiamine, mg.	1.0	1.2
Riboflavin, mg.	1.2	1.7
Vitamin C, mg.	30	70

Minerals

Minerals are inorganic elements (i.e., derived from nonliving sources) which, like vitamins, are vital to body functioning in very small amounts. Currently known are eight essential minerals and six trace elements.

Calcium and phosphorus, plentiful in milk and green leafy vegetables, provide the structure of bones and teeth. Iodine affects the thyroid gland. Goiter is a mineral deficiency disease, which we prevent by adding a trace of iodine to table salt (iodized salt) in areas where foods naturally containing iodine, such as ocean fish, are not generally consumed.

Iron affects the oxygen-carrying ability of the blood, and a deficiency of iron can cause anemia. This mineral is found in red meats, dark whole grains, green vegetables, and often in drinking water. One out of every four teenage and adult women is believed to be deficient in iron to some degree, symptomized by skin pallor and fatigue. In other eras, curiously, more traces of iron were found in food than are today because of the widespread use of iron cooking vessels in American homes.

Minerals, like vitamins, can be ingested as supplementary food pills. Except in specific instances (such as goiter and iron deficiency anemia) there remains considerable question whether mineral supplements are helpful, potentially harmful, or simply unnecessary. Warnings on the bottle to keep iron pills, etc., out of the reach of children testifies to the possible toxicity of large doses.

Water

Man consists of about 71 percent water by body weight, and water is involved in every physiological or chemical process of the human body. Water in the bloodstream carries nutrients to all organs and cells and removes the waste products. Altogether, it takes five to six pints of water to replace the daily losses in breathing, perspiration, and excretion.

Hence water is vital to body functions. A man may drink about three pints a day directly. He takes in another two pints with food (even the driest grains or crackers will contain some water). The body creates the rest of his six pints in the oxidation of food through digestion and metabolism—the same water-making phenomenon that causes an automobile exhaust to steam and a smoker's pipe to bubble.

It is virtually impossible to drink too much water; many people do not drink enough. One of the simplest cures for constipation, a common condition, is to drink four glasses of water a day in addition to any other liquid foods or beverages.

People seeking to lose weight often make the mistake of avoiding water because it "puts on pounds." In fact, water is retained in the body only as required by the tissues, and the balance is a very precise one. Fat people retain water because of the presence of the fat, not the other way around. One of the more spectacular results of a reducing diet that eliminates excess fatty tissues is a sudden loss of water as well. When loss of water and fat is excessive relative to intake, one may become dehydrated. This can occur during strenuous physical effort with profuse sweating, especially in hot weather, and may cause weakness, cramps or faintness. Such losses are readily replaced through drinking and eating.

Everything we consume contains some water which is beneficial but other ingredients are often overlooked as a source of calories. A glass of soda pop contains 70 to 100 calories (from the sugar), an eight-ounce glass of beer about 120 calories, four ounces of wine 80 to 120 calories, and a cocktail 180 to 220 calories. Hard liquors (whiskey, gin, vodka, rum, brandy) contain as many calories per ounce as the proof of the liquor; thus a jigger (1½ oz.) of Scotch (86 proof) contains about 130 calories even when diluted by water or soda. A cup of coffee with cream and sugar approximates 45 calories; black coffee, none.

The Four Food Groups

Some understanding of the nutritive value of foods is essential both in preparing proper meals at home and in choosing wisely from a menu at a restaurant. But it is not necessary to carry around calorie charts and a pocket calculator to keep track of every nutrient in minute detail. As a practical guide to the composition of an adequate diet, the U.S. Department of Agriculture has divided common foods into four basic groups, which are easy to remember.

Each group consists of food servings having similar nutritive values. Selection of foods as indicated in the table on pages 36–37 provides adequate amounts of important nutrients more or less automatically. One selection from each group each day will supply an adult with 50 to 70 percent of his daily calorie allowance, 80 percent of iron, 80 percent of thiamine, 90 percent of niacin, and 100 percent of riboflavin according to the Recommended Dietary Allowances (RDA). The remaining percentages of these nutrients, as well as others not mentioned in the table, are supplied by auxiliary items commonly present in the American diet, such as butter, margarine, cooking fats, salad dressing, sugar, desserts, jams and syrups, white bread or cake made of unenriched flour, soft drinks, beer, etc. Each listing in the table is one serving.

The Four Food Groups (USDA)

Milk Group: 2 cups or equivalent servings per day (3–4 for children)

    1 cup of whole milk = 160 calories

    1 cup of skim milk, buttermilk, non-fat dry milk = 90 calories

    1 cup of chocolate milk = 190 calories

    1 cup of whole milk yogurt = 150 calories, reduced to 125 for skim yogurt, increased to 250 with sweetened fruit

    1 cup custard = 105 calories

    1 slice (1 ounce) Swiss cheese = 105 calories

    ½ cup cream cottage cheese = 130 calories

Fruit and Vegetable Group: 4 servings per day

    Rich in Vitamin C: Citrus fruits or juice; cantaloupe; papaya; strawberries; tomatoes or juice; Brussels sprouts; broccoli

    Rich in Vitamin A: (Deep yellow) carrots; pumpkin; sweet potato; winter squash; cantaloupe; apricots. (Dark green) collard greens, kale, mustard greens, spinach, turnip greens

    6 ounces unsweetened fruit juice = 80 calories

    ½ banana or grapefruit = 40 calories

    1 cantaloupe = 30 calories

    1 peach, pear, apple, orange = 80 calories

    1 cup canned fruit = 40 calories (no sugar) to 100 calories (heavy syrup)

    ½ cup potatoes, corn, lima beans = 70 calories

    ½ cup beets, carrots, onions, peas, squash = 35 calories

    ½ cup leafy greens, green cooked vegetables, eggplant, celery, tomatoes, etc. = 20 calories

Meat Group: 2 servings per day = 5 ounces

    2–3 ounces* fish or shellfish meat = 100 to 200 calories

    2–3 ounces* poultry meat = 90 to 200 calories

    2–3 ounces* cooked lean meat = 120 to 175 calories

    1 hamburger = 245 calories

    2 eggs = 160 calories

    2–3 ounces hard cheese = 230 calories

    *Not counting bones, skin, fat, or shells.

Alternates:
1 cup cooked dried beans, peas, lentils = 200 calories
½ cup nutmeats = 400 calories
⅓ cup peanuts = 280 calories
4 tablespoons peanut butter = 380 calories
Bread and Cereal Group: 4 servings per day**
1 slice bread = 65 calories
½ cup cooked cereal = 60 calories
1 roll, biscuit, muffin = 100 calories
1 cup (1 ounce) dry cereal, plain = 110 calories
½ cup cooked pasta (spaghetti, noodles, etc.) = 100 calories
**All grain foods should be made with whole-grain or enriched flour.

Milk Group

The milk group provides protein of excellent quality and in abundant quantity, as well as calcium, riboflavin, fat, and several other items. Milk has sometimes been called (incorrectly) "the perfect food," since it contains significant amounts of most nutrients required by man except iron, and smaller amounts of vitamins A, C, and D. It is not quite perfect, however. Infants can thrive on an exclusive milk diet, but demand an increasing variety of foods as they grow.

Adults should drink milk *as a food,* not as a beverage like water added to food intake. It contains too many calories and too much fat to ignore. For practical purposes one may freely interchange whole milk, buttermilk, skim milk, or cottage cheese in composing a diet. Hard cheeses and ice cream may also be considered milk equivalents. If you don't drink milk, physicians may recommend a calcium supplement (mineral pill).

Fruits and Vegetables

The fruit and vegetable group includes the sources of 60 percent of vitamin A and 90 percent of vitamin C in the average diet, and lesser sources of riboflavin, thiamine, calcium, iron, and folic acid. Surveys indicate that vitamin C is the vitamin most often found lacking in the typical diet, while vitamin A often is in short supply among the elderly.

These omissions are easily rectified by one serving a day of a C food and at least one every other day of an A food.

Fruits and vegetables also provide some carbohydrate and—quite important—fiber and bulk. They contain much water and in this respect are the exact opposite of highly concentrated foods like sugar, flour, or cheese. One can nibble on a raw carrot or a stalk of celery as a snack without concern about calories. The fibrous bulk fills the stomach and promotes the peristaltic action of the intestines.

There is much talk about organically grown fruits and vegetables being more natural and therefore more nutritious. In actual fact, one can accomplish more nutritionally by better cooking methods. Cook vegetables as little as possible, in as small an amount of water as possible, and save the cooking water for soups and sauces. The experts on this technique are the Chinese.

Breads and Cereals

Grains and grain products provide a highly acceptable source of calories—the basic energy food of mankind since the invention of agriculture—along with B vitamins, protein, and iron. In fact, it is difficult to obtain a sufficient quantity of thiamin, riboflavin, niacin, and iron if this group of carbohydrates is excluded from the diet.

Be wary of prejudice against bread as a "fattening food." One ounce of cooked, sliced roast beef has 73 calories, while a slice of bread has only 68 calories. This means that a person can eat more meat than he needs *or* more bread than he needs and add pounds; and he can add extra calories to either by not trimming the fat on the meat or adding gravy, or by putting butter on his bread. Obviously no single food is fattening; body fat accumulates only when total calorie intake exceeds caloric consumption. The change in the American diet to more highly refined grain products and refined sugar has been related to the high incidence of dental decay and increases in cancer of the colon and the intestines. More emphasis needs to be placed on eating whole-grain products and less baked products high in sugar. For example, eating plain oatmeal rather than a sweetened cereal is a better choice for breakfast.

Nutritionally speaking, a white bread enriched with vitamins and minerals is *similar* to whole-grain bread, except that the latter contains more bulk (bran). This is why the four servings per day specified in the bread and cereals group of a balanced diet preferably should be whole-grain products.

The Meat Group

The meat group includes all food from land animals and fish, including eggs, plus dried legumes (beans, peas) and nuts. The latter foods may be considered meat substitutes, since they are almost as good a source of edible protein. In addition, the meat group supplies vitamins of the B complex such as thiamine, riboflavin, niacin, and B_6, and iron. Variety (organ) meats are a good source of Vitamin B_{12}.

The dietary problem with meat is the fat it often contains, bringing calories and cholesterol to the body in rather large amounts. Even lean meat contains 5 to 10 percent fat, and the better the quality grade (prime, choice) the more the meat is marbled with fat. Fish contains very little fat, but a one-pound steak may contain four to five ounces of saturated fat. When you sit down to one of these beauties, your reward is 1,440 calories, or about half the total daily need, and 320 milligrams of cholesterol, or 20 milligrams more than the recommended maximum of 300—all in one dish!

Shellfish, organ meats, and eggs also are high in cholesterol; the heart patient's prudent diet limits him to two or three servings *per week*. The chart indicates five ounces of meat or *its equivalent* per day, which in turn could mean *smaller* portions of meat, eggs, etc., per serving and a *larger* proportion of meat protein equivalents.

Again we may gain a cue from traditional cookery: e.g., Yankee bean soup, Canadian pea soup, chili con carne with beans, Brazilian black beans and rice, and many other dishes from all over the world mingle legumes with small amounts of meat or with carbohydrates. Since meat is the largest element of cost in the food budget, learning to eat nutritionally from the food-group chart can save a lot of money, too.

In summary, learning a few facts about food—and disregarding the fads and fallacies—can play a major role in physical fitness. In the next chapter the relationship of calories to exercise will be explained.

Chapter 4

BE FIT, NOT FAT

In the previous chapter calories were defined not as a food or a nutrient but as a measure of energy. We take in calories (or energy) every time we eat and we expend calories (or energy) every moment we live: by every motion, even to take a breath or wink an eye, by the beating of the heart and in the process of digestion while we are asleep. The more active we are, the more calories we expend.

Excess calories mean excess weight. Hence there are two ways to control weight, one by taking in fewer calories each day, the other by expending more calories each day through physical activity. The relationship between the two is not much more complicated than simple arithmetic.

Here is a table comparing a number of foods—each equal to 100 calories—and a number of activities—each of which burns up 100 calories:

Plus 100 Calories	Minus 100 Calories
2 pats of butter or margarine	Walking 1½ miles
1⅔ tablespoons of honey	Jogging ¾ mile
2 tablespoons salted peanuts	Bicycling 2½ miles
2 slices bacon	Dancing 25 minutes
2 tablespoons whipped cream	Playing tennis 15 minutes
2¼ tablespoons sugar	Hand lawn-mowing 30 minutes
3⅓ tablespoons coffee cream	Horseback riding (trot) 20 minutes
¼ of a chocolate ice cream soda	Working 2 days in office
1½ slices white bread	132 push-ups
etc.	etc.

41

This list could be continued through hundreds of items, but the entries above make the point. It is easy to feed calories to the body but difficult to burn them up—e.g., a week and a half's office work equals 1 chocolate soda. One pound of body fat equals approximately 3,500 calories. Professor Arthur H. Steinhaus has pointed out that each pound of fat burned results in a weight loss of 1¼ to 1½ pounds because the body also releases water normally retained with the fat.

To some this sounds discouraging. To lose a pound of fat you would have to walk more than eleven hours, or swim more than five hours, or bicycle more than seven hours. Hence there is a myth popular among the overweight that exercise is not useful for losing poundage. It's a myth because you don't have to consider the exercise being performed in one unbearably exhausting ordeal.

Weight loss from intensified physical activity will come whether the exercise is done in a few hours or over the course of a year. For example, a pleasant half hour of bicycling every evening would total the desired seven hours in a couple of weeks. At that rate one could shed twenty-six pounds of body fat in one year.

Fitness vs. Fatness

An obese person worries about his fatness as an esthetic and social disadvantage. He would do better to worry about his unfitness, of which fatness is but one outward sign. If he were physically fit, he would probably not be fat. It is impossible to be in full bloom of health and at the same time overweight. In the case of an obese person, body conditioning might save his life.

The truth about calories is so simple that people somehow hate to admit it. If the number of calories ingested as food should correspond exactly to the number consumed in the metabolism, body weight would not change except for minor fluctuations in water content, up to about two pounds a day. But all excess calories eaten and not burned are converted into fat. This is nature's way, inherited from a period in man's evolution when starvation was always just around the corner, of storing food when it's plentiful for supplying energy another day when it's not.

It doesn't matter whether the calories ingested are in the form of fat, carbohydrates, or protein—from butter, bread, or beef—and neither does it matter how the calories are expended in the body or how long it takes. A person with a sedentary occupation and little physical activity during leisure might have an energy output representing about eleven ounces of fatty tissue per day. An athlete in training or a lumberman chopping down trees might expend the daily equivalent of two pounds of fatty tissue.

Most Americans tend to put on weight after the age of 25 because energy consumption does not keep pace with calorie input. In youth we acquire certain food habits, such as a desire for sweets, which appear to do us no harm *at that time* because we counterbalance the intake of calories with strenuous physical activity. But when physical activity declines with the passing years, following the selfsame food habits will make us fat.

Professor Per-Olof Astrand states as a rule of thumb that "a person's weight should not increase after his or her twenties. Since muscular tissue declines [with age] a loss of a few pounds is actually good proof [of] no increase in fatty tissue."

In other words, to stay fit weigh what you weighed in the twenties—or less!

Exercise and Appetite

The mechanism of appetite conspires to overfeed a sedentary person. In a healthy animal, including human beings, the appetite rises or falls naturally in tune with the body's need for energy output. You work, you play, you get hungry—it's as simple as that. But this appetite mechanism can go awry. Every mother knows how difficult a child can be when it refuses to eat. (The cure for "difficult eaters": just whisk the food away until the hungry child lets out a bellow.)

Dr. Jean Mayer of Harvard, perhaps America's top nutritionist, conducted appetite experiments with laboratory animals. When rats were exercised moderately, less than two hours a day, they did not eat more than unexercised rats; paradoxically, they ate somewhat less. When exercised more than two hours daily, putting extra energy demands upon the body, hunger was stimulated and they increased food intake to match the energy expenditure. This is the same mechanism of balancing input and output that can keep the weight of most human adults constant.

However, Dr. Mayer found that appetite failed to respond in proportion beyond a certain upper limit of exercise (i.e., approaching exhaustion), and it also failed to decrease when energy expenditure fell *below* a certain lower limit. The second finding is the important one in combating obesity. In an article on his findings in a Blue Cross publication, *Food & Fitness,* Dr. Mayer says: "The sedentary range is reached when one becomes so inactive that the appetite-regulating mechanism fails to lower food intake to match [lowered] energy expenditure." That is why sedentary rats ate more, not less than the moderately exercised rats—their energy output fell below the lower limit. A farmer seeking to fatten a pig or a steer knows what to do: he keeps the animal penned up and physically lazy while stuffing it with food.

Above this sedentary range of activity, appetite and exercise become attuned. Then appetite can be a sensitive and reliable regulator for matching food intake with energy outgo (if not carried to exhaustion). That's the way it was when manual labor was the way of life for average men and women. Since 1900, our average caloric intake has *decreased* while the prevalence of obesity has *increased*. We are fattening ourselves by defying a natural law.

Why We Put on Weight

Obesity only rarely stems from pathological or genetic disturbances. Fat children are simply less active than others. Programs involving hundreds of children have proved that even one hour of daily exercise could correct the fault. Inactivity also appears to be the main reason for obese adults, particularly males. What we now consider normally active, say two hours of walking every day and sports every weekend, would have been considered sedentary at the turn of the century.

With this habitual inactivity, the appetite regulator is often set for a calorie supply greater than the need. It would seem from the table on page 41 that restricting food intake offers the direct way out of the dilemma. But unfortunately there is no diet low enough in calories to reduce weight substantially and yet leave you satisfied. It is difficult to compose a low-calorie diet that also supplies a sufficient quantity of all the essential nutrients.

We therefore have an interesting choice. If we wish to lose weight, we can continue being habitually inactive but often uncomfortably hungry from dieting, or we can become moderately active and eat pretty much what we like.

If we take in only 50 kcal a day more than we need for energy output, which amounts to only about four teaspoons of sugar, we would end the year with a surplus of 18,250 kcal, or more than five pounds of fat. For the sake of a minor indulgence, we would put on fifty-two pounds in ten years!

Or, if we have routinely walked one mile each day, but then eliminate the walk without adjusting the diet, we could gain 100 pounds in ten years. That's why the approach of obesity is a stealthy one as years pass and one's lifestyle becomes more sedate. That's also why restoring the abandoned activity of youth is the key to curing obesity in middle age.

The sensible way to reduce weight involves taking plenty of time about it combined with persistence, the mirror image of the stealthy onslaught of obesity we have just described. You could eliminate 100 kcal a day from the diet just by drinking coffee black, without sugar and cream. You could burn up another 100 kcal with a one-and-a-half-mile walk each day. With these measures, other things being equal, the body statistically would hold 6,000 kcal less after one month, equivalent to about 1.7 pounds of fat. You'd lose about twenty pounds in a year! Just by taking a walk and drinking coffee black.

Crash Diets

As compared to this leisurely pace, a crash diet appears to do the same job virtually overnight. Unfortunately, crash diets are unhealthy and can even be dangerous. You are trying to get rid of excess fat because it puts a strain upon the body; a starvation regimen imposes even a greater strain. It lowers the resistance and leaves the body vulnerable to disease, fatigue, rapid aging, and other harmful effects.

To cut down on food intake to the point of starvation leads to loss of energy, loss of muscle tone, low endurance, and low reserves of the sustenance you need for work, sports, mental alertness, sex life—or any other activity. Diets based upon a single "magic" food, such as a grapefruit diet, high protein–low fat diet, cream diet, etc., have the drawback of being nutritionally inadequate. Thus a rice and fruit diet sounds good, but lacks some necessary amino acids, minerals, enzymes, and vitamins.

Diet and exercise go together. If you diet without exercising, the result may be a thin weak person in place of a fat weak person. Muscle tissue that is not used will atrophy and proportionately become fatter even though the intake of calories has been reduced.

On the other hand, if you exercise enough, you can pretty much ignore dieting except for certain minor restrictions that are simply common sense. Not only is the food you eat burned up, but its nutrients are absorbed more efficiently and carried to every cell in the active body. Note that professional athletes are big eaters, yet it does them no harm so long as they keep busy at the physical labor of their trade.

New Eating Patterns

The minor diet restrictions referred to above are readily effected and make it easier to gain benefit from exercise in your body conditioning program. What we outline here is *not* a diet, but a series of small adjustments in eating patterns.

If you carried around a notebook and wrote down everything you ate in the course of a day, every single potato chip, you might be appalled. The traditional "three square meals a day" of agricultural days have all but disappeared in urban life. We may be eating virtually continuously from dawn to dark. Let's see:

Breakfast has become a quick meal except on leisurely Sunday mornings. Traditional items such as eggs, bacon, or pancakes take too long to prepare when people are in a hurry to get to work or school, so they "grab" a fast breakfast of fruit juice, toast, and coffee, or corn flakes and milk, or an "instant" liquid meal that comes in a jar.

At work or in school there is always a break in the morning for food of some kind. A working adult may grab several cups of coffee between breakfast and lunch, sometimes with a sweet roll or a doughnut. Women do the same at home. Vending machines in factories, office buildings, schools tempt us constantly with soft drinks, candy bars, potato chips, coffee, crackers, and cookies.

Luncheon today is eaten "out" by most adults. Even if they carry a lunch box from home, they will almost surely supplement their sandwich with snacks and drinks. Meals served in lunchrooms are notoriously filling without much regard to nutriment, even in expensive places. Then there may be another coffee (and cake) break in midafternoon.

Dinner remains the one meal that Americans enjoy at leisure and still regard as a semi-formal occasion, even though served at home. But snacking may begin as soon as dinner is over. An entire line of packaged foods is referred to in the trade as "TV snacks."

When you ask people about their diet, they nearly always can tell you what they ate for dinner, the big meal of each day. They rarely remember to include the countless hot dogs, hamburgers, cakes, candies, coffees, beers, cheese crackers, Cokes, cocktails, salted peanuts, corn chips, pizza slices, etc., etc., they have grabbed on the run all day long.

Foods to Avoid

Snacking creates nutritional problems not so much from the constant nibbling (which is actually a more natural way to eat than in three formal meals a day), but from the "junk" foods that careless habits and indefatigable promotion have made into favorite snacks. By definition, a junk food is anything edible that contains little or no essential nutrients except calories, and one that replaces nutritionally more important foods.

Calories are necessary for energy; thus a candy bar could be a lifesaver for an exhausted soldier in a foxhole. It becomes a junk food if eaten by a child and replacing more wholesome foods containing proteins or other essential nutrients. In seeking physical fitness, you can help your cause by *discriminating* among foods nutritively.

Fats, sweets, and alcohol come in for much unfavorable attention because they contain a lot of calories concentrated into very little bulk. They are pleasant to take, easy to eat,

47

and tempting. Avoiding them keeps surplus calories out of the system and encourages an appetite for the bulkier foods that supply essential proteins and other nutrients.

Fats

A certain amount of fat will be present in virtually any meat you eat, also in breads or cakes prepared with shortening of any kind. Such foods should supply enough fat for any true nutritional purpose; any additional fat means just so many additional calories. Therefore it's a good idea to cut down on foods *to which fat has been deliberately added*, such as whipped cream toppings, the lard or shortening in pies and pastries, cream salad dressings, and all fried foods. It was a dark day for the obese when French-fried potatoes (in deep fat) replaced boiled potatoes (in the jackets) as the American favorite.

Excess fats are unwelcome whether saturated or unsaturated. In terms of calories, fat is fat. In terms of cholesterol, there may or may not be much net difference among types of fats in the diet. It is generally agreed that some fat in the diet is essential, even though the body manufactures its own fat out of carbohydrates and other foodstuffs in metabolizing them for the extraction of energy.

Reducing fat intake often amounts to changing one's taste in customary foods or learning new tricks of cookery. Here is a "prudent" version of a well-known dish:

Bacon and Egg

On half of a toasted English muffin place one slice of grilled Canadian bacon, and on the bacon place a poached egg. Sprinkle with fresh-ground pepper. Cut up together to eat.

On first reading that may sound like an orgy of cholesterol and calories, until you notice certain subtle modifications:

1. Half an English muffin, not a whole one.
2. Lean Canadian (back) bacon instead of fat slab (belly) bacon.
3. One egg, not two.

48

4. Egg cooked in water, not fried in fat.
5. No butter on the bread.
6. No salt on the egg.

You can eat this with relish and no sense of deprivation. This is not dieting, but it does represent a minor adjustment in habit to avoid too much fat, too many calories, too much salt, or eating too much just because it tastes good. When numerous dishes have been slightly modified for nutritional thrift, the saving in calories will mount to a surprising total in the course of a year.

Sugar

Another highly concentrated food, refined sugar, comes in for criticism as if there were something wrong with it intrinsically. There isn't, except for the calories packed into small space with no other minerals, vitamins, or nutrients of any description. A cube of sugar is pure carbohydrate, yet it seems to disappear and become nothing when dissolved in water. Excessive intake of sugar has been associated with dental caries, heart disease, stomach and bowel disorders, and cancer.

People drink soft drinks to quench their thirst without realizing they are ingesting calories as the sweetening. A chocolate bar is so rich with carbohydrate (sugar) and fat (cocoa butter) that the Army uses it for emergency rations. Honey, molasses, cane syrup, and other forms of sugar are just as rich as the refined variety, although they may contain traces of minerals as additional nutrients.

Instead of sweets, drink skimmed or low-fat milk, fruit juices, and plenty of water. Learn to enjoy the flavor of coffee or tea without sweetening; it will make a coffee and tea connoisseur of you. For snacks, turn to raisins, apples, carrots, celery. Keep unsweetened fruit juices in the refrigerator as thirst quenchers, partially diluted with ice or water. Cook dried fruits, such as prunes, without sugar. Here's a delicious recipe:

Natural Prunes

Fill a quart jar partway with dried prunes. Add a sprinkling of raisins. Add more prunes, more raisins, etc., in layers until jar is loosely filled. Put a slice of lemon on top. Fill the jar with boiling water. Cover. Let stand at room temperature 24 hours. Replace any absorbed liquid with more water. Refrigerate.

Some current research points the finger of suspicion at too much sugar in the diet, rather than too much fat, as the basis of cholesterol in the blood. Whatever the exact chemistry may be, there's no doubt that *unneeded calories* taken into the system too quickly and easily in concentrated foods *of any kind* are not conducive to physical fitness.

Salt

Nutritionally, many if not most people eat too much salt. This mineral, sodium chloride, is essential to human life and was a precious commodity in early societies. The word *salary* stems from a Roman custom of paying troops in rations of salt (*sal*). The sodium in the compound is the significant element; it occurs naturally in a number of food plants; but our chief source of it is common salt.

The water in the human body is maintained at a precise level of salinity, which is maintained by balancing salt intake and loss with freshwater intake and loss. When this balance is upset, the body suffers. Thus an abrupt salt loss caused by heavy perspiration may cause weakness, which is readily relieved by increasing the salt intake. Too much salt, on the other hand, makes one thirsty for a greater intake of water.

The typical daily sodium intake may be about 3,000 milligrams. This can be cut in half, with no nutritional loss, simply by refraining from adding salt to foods as served at the table. Practically all prepared foods (e.g., baker's bread) contain some salt, added for the sake of flavor, and salt may be present in meat or milk. Elimination of heavily salted foods, such as smoked meat and fish, or condiments, such as pickles, offers another way to cut down.

A large sodium intake is directly related to certain types of high blood pressure and cardiovascular and kidney disease.

With these conditions a physician might prescribe a diuretic to rid the body of retained excess water; the presence of salt acts in just the opposite way to retain water in the body. In middle age, going easy on the salt is a simple, practical way to head off some of these troubles. Again, this is accomplished by a change in taste favoring the true flavor of a food over added saltiness. A low-sodium or completely sodium-free diet, if prescribed by a physician, can be tolerated by learning to enjoy herbs and spices to give flavor to food without salt.

All table salt is the same nutritionally, although there may be differences in taste. Those who consider variations such as sea salt or coarse rock salt to be more healthful are really talking about impurities in the product rather than the salt itself. These impurities conceivably could include other minerals of some nutritional value. But sodium is sodium regardless of whether the salt has been refined, treated for smooth pouring, iodized, evaporated, or crudely chopped out of a rock and crushed.

Taste a dish before adding salt (then don't add it); it will make the cook happy and could help preserve your good health.

Smoking

Warning: The Surgeon General Has Determined That Cigarette Smoking Is Dangerous to Your Health

This grim legend was placed by law on all American cigarette packages about ten years ago, when there were 50 million smokers. Today there are 52 million. About 10 million Americans have managed to give it up, but a million new smokers, male and female, enter the ranks each year. A strange statistic! There is simply no question that smoking is a killer habit. From the point of view of physical fitness, tobacco is a curse.

Three elements in tobacco smoke are poisonous: nicotine, tar, and carbon monoxide. The nicotine and the carbon monoxide are pathologically related to heart and artery diseases. The tar collects in the pulmonary passages, opening the way to emphysema and cancer. These facts are not disputed. Yet habitual smoking continues to be an element of diet, or daily intake, that must be reckoned with, and a devilish habit to quit.

Nicotine is a subtle poison; 60 milligrams by mouth can cause death. One filter cigarette may contain 20 to 30 milligrams of nicotine of which the smoker inhales one or two. Even on that much, the blood pressure rises, the pulse quickens, the heart rate increases, the peripheral blood vessels contract, and the skin slightly chills. Most of these direct effects last about half an hour—which appears to be why the victim of the habit continually craves another cigarette.

In the nervous system, nicotine acts as a stimulant, then as a depressant. But its exact action upon the metabolism is not fully understood, except that *something* happens in the course of building up a tolerance for nicotine that enforces the addiction. Most likely it is a psychological addiction. The withdrawal symptoms are not fully dissipated by nicotine injections. Over the course of years, the physical damage can be very severe.

Carbon monoxide, the same gas that makes an automobile exhaust lethal in a closed area, is a product of combustion, and a smoker inhales a lot of it. Recent evidence of its cardiac effects on smokers has been published by the American Heart Association. Experimental animals exposed to carbon monoxide for several months show changes in the arterial walls that look exactly like atherosclerosis, along with degenerative changes in the heart muscle (myocardium).

Carbon monoxide does its damage by replacing oxygen in hemoglobin, the substance in the blood that carries oxygen from the lungs to the cells of the body. The myocardium is especially sensitive to oxygen deprivation. When this tissue suffocation is added to the effect of nicotine in constricting the blood vessels and further interfering with oxygen circulation, the result can be—sudden death.

Life insurance statistics demonstrate that the life expectancy of an individual 50 years of age is cut by eight and one-half years if he has smoked a pack of cigarettes a day for thirty years. Any number of other studies have found the same correlation: don't smoke and you live longer.

It is difficult to convince people that smoking is dangerous until some compelling event—such as a heart attack—makes the truth clear. The habit takes many years to wreak its slow but murderous damage. Physiological problems may not come home to roost until one's fifties or sixties, when the incidence of heart disease, arteriosclerosis, emphysema, and lung cancer begins climbing at a frightening pace.

Athletes in training don't smoke. Men and women interested in physical fitness don't smoke. They feel and perform better without it.

A recent newsletter of the Vanderbilt Branch YMCA in New York, written by René Biourd, Physical Director, contained this intriguing item:

MORE ABOUT TOBACCO . . .
Another aspect of the damages brought about by smoking is that it has an inhibiting effect on sexual drive. A. Ochusner reports: "It has been surprising to me the number of heavy smoking patients and friends, having discontinued smoking for health and other reasons, who have volunteered one of the greatest advantages of the discontinuance of tobacco has been the unexpected increase in libido."
Is not this an incentive to quit? Right away?

Chapter 5

YOUR IDEAL WEIGHT

As a starting point toward body conditioning, the first step nearly always is a step on to a scale. Body weight, especially overweight, offers the most obvious symptom that some sort of conditioning program would be a good idea, and how far it should go. Probably the majority of adult Americans are overweight to some degree, and at least 20 percent are definitely obese.

"Nobody loves a fat man," intones the old saying. Women seem to feel that the aphorism goes double for them. American women are the world's most enthusiastic dieters, hoping to shed excess pounds for the sake of better appearance. When they succeed, generally they should also enjoy better health.

The medical definition of obesity has undergone refinement in recent years, but by consensus among physiologists it means any person who is more than 10 to 20 percent heavier than his or her ideal weight. Such unsightly girth poses a formidable barrier to physical fitness as well as to social success.

A very heavy person punishes the vital organs of the body just by dragging around all that extra flesh. Pounds of fat have to be supplied with blood, oxygen, nutrients, and waste disposal by a heart, lung, liver, kidney, etc., which nature designed for a smaller body. In the United States today, obesity is well recognized as a direct hazard to health. Being too fat is related to the incidence of coronary heart disease, diabetes, cirrhosis of the liver, and various mechanical failures of body structure or function, such as hernia, lower back pain, flat feet, and intestinal obstruction.

On the Scale

If good physical condition is related to a person's weight, ascertaining the ideal weight for that person becomes a highly important consideration. One's gross weight as measured directly on the scale does not tell the whole story. Common charts and tables of the "average weight" of men and women according to height in inches provide only a rough approximation. Such averages were worked out early in this century by insurance companies who simply weighed all applicants for their policies. The figures are inadequate as a guide for a number of reasons.

By definition, an average is the sum of a group of values divided by the number of values. If one person weighs 175 pounds and a second person 125 pounds, then their average weight is $\dfrac{175 + 125}{2} = \dfrac{300}{2} = 150$ pounds. Obviously this kind of average summarizes a broad range of values, a range of 50 pounds from 125 to 175 in the example. If we wanted to determine the physiologically correct weight for either of the two individuals, the average would not be particularly instructive.

About thirty years ago the significance of wide deviations from a mathematical average weight was recognized by classifying body build or morphology into three types. The *endomorphic* type has a body structure tending to largeness; the *ectomorphic* has a lean build; and the *mesomorphic* has a triangular, muscular build.

It is possible for a mesomorph to weigh more than average without being obese. For example, if a man five feet eight inches tall weighed 160 pounds, he would be in the acceptable range if he had a large frame—although he would be 10 to 20 pounds overweight with a medium frame, and 20 to 30 pounds overweight with a small frame. Consequently the target or ideal weight of a body conditioning program would be entirely different for each individual.

In modern physical testing, it is conceded that gross weight may be a misleading measure. More scientific methods are currently in use at the YMCA and by physicians. These endeavor to determine the *body composition*. Whatever the total weight may be, how much of the body is lean and how much of it is fat?

Estimating Body Composition

One's lean body weight (LBW) is the key figure. Knowing the LBW, we can subtract it from gross body weight to find the weight of fat in the body. The percentage of fat—the ratio of fat to lean—specifies the category of body composition. This in turn makes possible a calculation of ideal weight for the individual whether ecto-, endo-, or mesomorphic.

The most accurate method of estimating body composition was invented more than two thousand years ago by the Greek mathematician Archimedes, who sought a way to determine the percent of base metal in an alloy of gold. Pondering the problem one day in the public bath, he observed the displacement of water by his immersed body.

Archimedes realized that the volume of water displaced would equal the volume of the object displacing it. With that information he could determine the density of the gold alloy—its weight per unit of volume—and thereby how much of it was pure gold.

The inspiration so excited Archimedes that he dashed from the bath and ran home naked through the streets shouting, "Eureka ("I have found it)!" In shortcut form, Archimedes' principle is still employed in hydrostatic weighing. An object is weighed, then weighed again under water, where it appears to weigh less. The difference is the weight of water displaced, from which the volume displaced is readily calculated.

Since hydrostatic weighing involves a rather awkward dousing when the object to be weighed is a living person, other means have been found that utilize key measurements of the body. The estimated weight is useful in programming one's physical activity, and much more significant than gross weight taken alone. Some of these methods, including one which a person can use on himself, are described in this chapter.

What Fat Estimates Mean

From the standpoint of good health, a male should probably have less than 20 percent fat in his total body weight. If good looks are his aim, he should weigh in at less than 16 percent fat. For the trim, hard body of an athlete, 10 percent fat should be the upper limit. The target in physical fitness work generally considers 16 percent fat good.

At the opposite extreme, any male who possesses an excess of 30 percent fat would certainly be considered obese—in fact, a medical problem. Here are normal percentages for degrees of physical fitness as worked out by measuring middle-aged males and adjusting the scale for women:

PERCENT FAT IN BODY COMPOSITION

		Men	Women
Very Lean	Excellent	8–10%	8–11%
Lean	Good	12–14%	13–16%
Average	Average	16–20%	18–22%
Fat	Fair	22–24%	24–27%
Very Fat	Poor	26–28%	29–32%

Any person of any age whose body composition places him in the *fair* or *poor* category of the table, that is, one whose proportion of fat in the body exceeds 20 to 30 percent, should take warning. Health hazards abound. Practically all work or exertion is difficult for this person because of the obesity, and exercise must be tailored to his ability to tolerate it. He or she should consult a doctor to prescribe a diet in combination with a carefully modified program of exercise, designed to bring his weight within at least the *average* range of body fat percentages within a reasonable time.

Note that this is no recommendation for a crash diet. There simply is no safe way to lose weight overnight. The pounds lost quickly by a crash diet usually do not stay lost. A realistic goal for a body conditioning diet provides 500 fewer calories per day than normal maintenance, and the reducing diet is continued only as long as necessary to attain the target weight. (See Chapter 4 for more about weight loss and diets.)

Quick Skinfold Test

You can find out when a person is not just "fat" but truly obese with a test that takes only a moment. Simply pinch the skin on the back of the upper arm. If the fold or pinched skin on a man's arm is one inch thick or more, the man is definitely obese. For a woman the critical measurement is one and one-half inches.

The rationale of skinfold measuring is that the pinched area enfolds only fat lying just beneath the skin, not the underlying muscle tissue. The wider the skinfold, the thicker the layer of subcutaneous fat not only at that spot but everywhere in the body. The inch- or inch-and-a-half arm thicknesses just described have been found by research to be reliable indicators that 30 percent of the person's body weight is adipose, fatty tissue. A glance at the table on page 58 shows that this degree of obesity would be rated poor or worse—out of the fit class altogether.

Similar correlationships have been established between fat weight and readily measured body structures such as parts of the skeleton or a protruding abdomen. Some of these tests use special calipers or other technical devices which should be left to trained hands, although described later in this chapter. However, you can make a reasonably accurate estimate of body composition with only two simple measurements—body weight and waist girth—requiring no special equipment or technique.

Measuring Yourself

The equation for this anthropometric test was developed in 1969 by J. H. Wilmore and A. T. Behnke from study of a group of young men. It has since been found applicable as well to the middle-aged males whose norms are given in the table on page 58. To make this test, proceed as follows:

1. Using an accurate scale, find your nude body weight to the nearest pound.

2. With a tape measure, find your waist girth. Hold the tape measure perfectly horizontal at a level just below the navel.

3. Measure the waist girth several times. The relationship to physical condition of a "belly" or of "middle-age spread" may seem pretty obvious, but for program testing purposes it should be as accurately measured as possible. The measured values should be within plus or minus 1 percent if they are

DETERMINATION OF IDEAL BODY WEIGHT

Actual Body Weight

Percent Fat	120	125	130	135	140	145	150	155	160	165	170	175	180	185	190	195	200	205	210	215	220	225	230	235	240
.6	134	140	145	151	157	162	168	173	179	185	190	196	201	207	213	218	224	229	235	241	246	252	257	263	269
.8	131	137	142	148	153	159	164	170	175	181	186	192	197	203	208	214	219	225	230	235	241	246	252	257	263
10	129	134	139	145	150	155	161	166	171	177	182	188	193	198	204	209	214	220	225	230	236	241	246	252	257
12	126	131	136	141	147	152	157	162	168	173	178	183	189	194	199	204	210	215	220	225	230	236	241	246	251
14	123	128	133	138	143	148	154	159	164	169	174	179	184	189	195	200	205	210	215	220	225	230	235	241	246
16	120	125	130	135	140	145	150	155	160	165	170	175	180	185	190	195	200	205	210	215	220	225	230	235	240
18	117	122	127	132	137	142	146	151	156	161	166	171	176	181	185	190	195	200	205	210	215	220	225	229	234
20	114	119	124	129	133	138	143	148	152	157	162	167	171	176	181	186	190	195	200	205	210	214	219	224	229
22	111	116	121	125	130	135	139	144	149	153	158	163	167	172	176	181	186	190	195	200	204	209	214	218	223
24	109	113	118	122	127	131	136	140	145	149	154	158	163	167	172	176	181	185	190	195	199	204	208	213	217
26	106	110	115	119	123	128	132	137	141	145	150	154	159	163	167	172	176	181	185	189	194	198	203	207	211
28	103	107	111	116	120	124	129	133	137	141	146	150	154	159	163	167	171	176	180	184	189	193	197	201	206
.30	100	104	108	113	117	121	125	129	133	138	142	146	150	154	158	163	167	171	175	179	183	188	192	196	200
32	97	101	105	109	113	117	121	125	130	134	138	142	146	150	154	158	162	166	170	174	178	182	186	190	194
34	94	98	102	106	110	114	118	122	126	130	134	138	141	145	149	153	157	161	165	169	173	177	181	185	189
36	91	95	99	103	107	110	114	118	122	126	130	133	137	141	145	149	152	156	160	164	168	171	175	179	183
38	89	92	96	100	103	107	111	114	118	122	125	129	133	137	140	144	148	151	155	159	162	166	170	173	177
40	86	89	93	96	100	104	107	111	114	118	121	125	129	132	136	139	143	146	150	154	157	161	164	168	171

On the left axis locate the estimated percent fat and on the horizontal axis locate the subject's actual body weight. The "ideal weight" (lean body weight plus 15% fat) is found at the intersection of these two variables.

to be significant. Using the two closest measurements, take the average and record this value to the nearest half inch.

4. Calculate the lean body weight (LBW) from the Wilmore-Behnke equation (below) or to simplify the arithmetic, use the conversion table (page 62).

5. Subtract the LBW from actual nude body weight. This gives the fat weight in pounds.

6. Divide fat weight by nude body weight to find the percent of fat in body composition.

7. From the table on page 60, determine the ideal weight for you. To use this table, you need only two factors: actual body weight (step 1) and percent fat (step 6).

Finally, compare your percent fat from this test to the norms for middle-aged persons on page 58, which will give you an idea where to set the objectives of your body conditioning program.

Wilmore-Behnke Equation

Given body weight in pounds and waist girth in inches, the lean body weight can be calculated from the following equation:

$$
\begin{aligned}
LBW = \ & 1.082 \text{ x body weight (lbs.)} \\
& - 4.15 \text{ x waist girth (in.)} \\
& + 98.42 \text{ (a constant)}
\end{aligned}
$$

To avoid most of the arithmetic, the conversion table on page 62 lists the numerical results when body weight is multiplied by 1.082 and waist girth is multiplied by 4.15. It is then an easy matter to add and subtract these conversion values and add the constant (98.42). Try this example:

Suppose a man weighs in at 176 pounds and the tape measure gives him a waist girth of 35 inches. In the conversion table we find the nearest values to 176 pounds and 35 inches and put down the matching conversion factors for our calculation.

CONVERSION FACTORS

Body Weight	cf	Waist Girth	cf
100	108.20	25.0	103.75
105	113.61	25.5	105.83
110	119.02	26.0	107.90
115	124.43	26.5	109.98
120	129.84	27.0	112.05
125	135.25	27.5	114.13
130	140.66	28.0	116.20
135	146.07	28.5	118.28
140	151.48	29.0	120.35
145	156.89	29.5	122.43
150	162.30	30.0	124.50
155	167.71	30.5	126.58
160	173.12	31.0	128.65
165	178.53	31.5	130.73
170	183.94	32.0	132.80
175	189.36	32.5	134.88
180	194.76	33.0	136.95
185	200.17	33.5	139.03
190	205.58	34.0	141.10
195	210.99	34.5	143.18
200	216.40	35.0	145.25
205	221.81	35.5	147.33
210	227.22	36.0	149.40
215	232.63	36.5	151.48
220	238.04	37.0	153.55
225	243.45	37.5	155.63
230	248.86	38.0	157.70
235	254.27	38.5	159.78
240	259.68	39.0	161.85
245	265.09	39.5	163.93
250	270.50	40.0	166.00

	Actual Measure	Conversion Factor
Weight 176 lbs.		189.36
Girth 35 in.		— 145.25
		44.11
Constant		+ 98.42
Lean body weight (LBW)		142.53 lbs.

To find the fat weight, subtract LBW from body weight.

Body weight	176.00 lbs.
LBW	— 142.53 lbs.
Fat weight	33.47 lbs.

Now find the percentage of fat in the body; divide fat weight by body weight and multiply by 100.

$$\frac{33.47}{176} = 0.190 \times 100 = 19.0 \text{ percent fat}$$

At his present weight of 176 pounds this man is 19 percent fat, which is somewhat higher than the ideal body composition of 16 percent fat. To find his ideal weight (i.e., what he would weigh if he were 16 percent fat), use the table on page 60.

The vertical scale of the table shows the estimated percent fat while the horizontal scale shows the measured body weight. Draw a straight line into the table from each of these two variables. The ideal weight (LBW + 16 percent) is located at the intersection of the two lines.

In the example given, we interpolate between 171 pounds at 18 percent fat and 167 pounds at 20 percent fat to determine the ideal weight for this 19 percent fat individual to be about 169 pounds.

Note: The mathematically minded can achieve somewhat greater precision than the table by using a simple formula:

$$\frac{\text{Fat weight x 16}}{\text{Percent fat}} = \text{Ideal fat weight in pounds}$$

Add the result to LBW from the earlier calculation to compute ideal total body weight for the individual. Substituting values for the above example, we get:

$$\frac{33.47 \times 16}{19} = \text{28.18 lbs. ideal fat weight}$$

$$+ \text{ 142.53 LBW}$$

$$= \text{170.71 lbs. ideal body weight}$$

The same equation may be used for establishing weight targets other than the 16 percent ideal conformation. If the 176-pound man in our example wants to train down to an athletic 10 percent fat, substitute 10 for 16 in the equation. This gives him:

$$\frac{33.47 \times 10}{19} = \text{17.61 fat weight}$$

$$+ \text{ 142.53 LBW}$$

$$= \text{160.14 lbs. athletic body weight}$$

Professional Body Measuring

The individual who joins a group physical fitness program such as an exercise class at the "Y" may find the physical director using even more sophisticated anthropometrics (body measurement). Research has developed a number of equations for body composition derived from measures of muscular girth, skinfolds, and skeletal diameters. The equations apply to specific groups—young or old, males or females, active or sedentary—and may not be applied to everyone indiscriminately.

One such equation uses waist girth (size), pectoral skinfold (fat), and wrist diameter (bone), all determined to fairly close tolerances for accuracy. While one's girth may be measured with an ordinary tape measure, the tape should be positioned carefully on the iliac crest (just above the hipbone) with the subject standing relaxed.

The pectoral skinfold is taken by pinching the flesh just between the left nipple and the shoulder and measuring its thickness with a specially designed skinfold caliper.

The wrist diameter is measured with a sliding caliper on the two outside bones, taking what is anatomically described as "the greatest distance between the styloid processes at the distal ends of the radius and ulna."

The equation used with these measures to estimate percent of fat in active adult males will be of interest if you undergo any of these scientific methods of modern physiological testing.

Percent fat = 8.7075 + 0.489 x waist girth (cm.)
+ 0.449 x pectoral skinfold (mm.)
− 6.359 x wrist diameter (cm.)

Another professional method takes a number of skinfold measurements to identify specific locations of fat deposits. A woman trying to reduce thick thighs may be more interested in fat on the thighs than in the body composition in general. For such tests the calipers are applied to skinfolds on the chest, the back of the arm, the lower tip of the shoulder blade, on the hip bone, just to the right or left of the navel, and on the front of the thigh.

These measurements in millimeters are then compared to a table of norms as shown below. In this way the progress of a fitness program can be charted precisely at particular parts of the body more accurately than from changes in percent of fat in the body as a whole.

SKINFOLD NORMS (Millimeters)

	Chest	Arm	Back	Hip	Abdomen	Thigh
Excellent	2	4	2	2	6	4
	5	5	5	5	8	6
Good	8	6	8	8	10	8
	11	7	11	11	14	10
Average	14	8	14	14	18	12
	17	9	17	17	22	14
	20	11	20	21	27	17
Fair	23	13	23	25	32	20
	26	15	26	29	37	23
Poor	28	17	29	33	42	26
	32	19	32	37	47	29

Chapter 6

THE PHYSIOLOGY OF EXERCISE

In recent years the question of exactly what happens in the body as the result of exercise has become a major concern of medical research. Interest has been stimulated by taking a new approach to the treatment of heart disease. While not denying the great strides that have been made in saving the victims of heart attacks, such as open heart surgery, it is now suspected that physical remedies, including exercise, can save just as many of the damaged circulatory systems as the surgery.

A 1974 forum sponsored by the American Heart Association assessed the results of coronary bypass surgery. In this dramatic operation, costing five or six thousand dollars, a section of a leg vein is transplanted in order to restore circulation to a dying heart muscle. The surgery, if successful, circumvents diseased coronary blood vessels and brings miraculous relief from the crushing pains of angina pectoris. But what of the patient's future? Will he be safer from dangerous heart attack after surgery?

The forum heard reports on three studies involving hundreds of patients at the University of Oregon School of Medicine, in veterans' hospitals, and in another group of hospitals. Preliminary results of these continuing studies found *no significant difference* in death rate or in the incidence of heart attack three years after the surgery. In the Oregon study, headed by Dr. J. David Bristow, cardiac sufferers not subjected to the operation had fared just as well as those who underwent surgery.

The control (non-operated) group of patients received the modern standard treatment for angina. The components of this standard treatment combine pharmaceutical with physical therapy in a revealing way:

- Nitroglycerine tablets to relieve the pain of angina.
- Drugs to reduce fats and cholesterol in the blood.
- Diet to reduce fats and cholesterol.
- Diet to control weight or eliminate obesity.
- No smoking.
- Regulated exercise.

The role of exercise in correcting cardiovascular problems or in preventing them in the first place is part of the complex science of exercise physiology. The balance of this chapter presents current responses to frequently asked questions as published in *The Y's Way to Physical Fitness,* edited by Myers, Sinning, Golding, 1973.

The Heart and Circulation

Q: *Is a low heart rate a good indicator of physical fitness when the pulse is taken at rest?*

A: The normal resting rate of the heart beat can range anywhere from forty to more than ninety beats per minute. A trained, extremely fit athlete such as a swimmer or track star will often have a slow heart rate, which in his case does indicate exceptional cardiac efficiency. But in sedentary people a slow heart does not necessarily indicate physical fitness; on the contrary, it may indicate some abnormality. Thus a carotid sinus syndrome (pressure on the carotid artery in the neck caused by arteriosclerosis) slows the heart beat by reflex action.

Training does result in a slower resting heart rate, but the decrease is not directly related to the degree of physical fitness. In any case, a resting heart rate cannot be determined by a single pulse; measurements should be taken over a period of several days to assure obtaining a true base value.

Q: *What is the maximum heart rate?*

A: During any exertion, including exercise, the heart rate or pulse speeds up. A maximum (or terminal) heart rate is the fastest heart beat that one may elicit during exercise, and exceeding it can be dangerous. As one grows older, the maximum heart rate decreases. The rule of thumb is to subtract age in years from 220 beats per minute. Thus for a man or woman of 40 the estimated maximum would be 180 beats per minute, at age 50 it would be 170, etc. In physical fitness programming, a participant's maximum heart rate is determined by preliminary tests.

Q: *What is the desirable training effect on the heart rate?*

A: A training effect is achieved by deliberately over-loading the body with physical exertion in order to improve conditioning and build up stamina. It is agreed among experts that the work load (for well individuals) must be sufficient to increase the heart rate during exercise by 60 percent toward the maximum rate; i.e., not all the way up to maximum, but 60 percent of the way. Thus the desired heart rate during exercise can be computed as:

Exercise rate = resting heart rate

+ .60 × (maximum heart rate — resting heart rate)

This derived rate is used to determine how intensive a person's exercise program should be.

Q: *What is the steady state of the heart beat?*

A: When exercising begins, a person's heart rate increases rapidly at first, then slowly for three to five minutes. It then levels off and remains quite constant during the remainder of the exercise. This level is the steady state of the heart rate. It has two uses:

If the exercise continues for a long period of time, a secondary rise above the steady state signals approaching exhaustion. The steady state also has value in testing and as a measure of work intensity during exercise.

Other physiological responses such as breathing and oxygen consumption reach a steady state during exercise very much like the heart rate.

Q: *What is the significance of the recovery heart rate?*

A: At the cessation of exercise, the heart rate begins to return toward resting values. The speed of recovery reflects the efficiency of the circulatory system. Faster recovery is one of the desired training effects.

The intensity of exercise affects recovery rate; so do temperature and other modifying factors. The heart rate during the *first fifteen seconds* following exercise is almost the same as the heart rate during the exertion and can be used as an indicator of exercise intensity.

Q: *Are all types of exercise good for the heart?*

A: Not necessarily. The person seeking cardiovascular improvement should select rhythmic, isotonic, or dynamic exercises such as walking, jogging, swimming, cycling, and certain calisthenics.

Isometric or static exercise and heavy weight lifting accelerate the heart by a reflex action, while at the same time developing a high resistance to blood flow and restricting venous return (return of blood to the heart). As a consequence, blood pressure rises unusually high relative to heart rate, with a possible reduction of the oxygen supply to the heart. A person who has or is susceptible to coronary heart disease should use such "strength-building" exercises with caution or avoid them altogether.

Rhythmic exercises tend to increase the heart rate without adversely raising the blood pressure. This is apparently due to the pumping action of the muscles returning the blood to the heart and lesser restriction of blood flow through the muscles than in static exercise. Since the heart rate increase comes in response to the body's demand for oxygen rather than to a nervous reflex, dynamic exercise is more effective than isometric exercise in improving cardiovascular efficiency.

Q: *What about blood pressure?*

A: Blood pressure is the force of the blood pushing against the walls of the arteries under the pumping action of the heart. Systolic pressure is the force developed when the heart contracts, while diastolic pressure is the force remaining in the arteries when the heart ends its relaxation phase and starts a new contraction. Pulse pressure is the difference between systolic and diastolic, the higher and lower of the two measures.

Blood pressure is measured with a sphygmomanometer. Air is pumped into a cuff placed around the upper arm at approximately heart level, which closes the brachial artery along the inside of the arm. The air then is allowed to escape slowly from the cuff. The pressure still remaining in the cuff at the moment the artery begins to push blood past it is equal to the systolic pressure. It is signaled by a distinctive loud "lub" sound picked up from the artery by listening through a stethoscope.

As air pressure in the cuff is further reduced, blood begins to flow through even while the heart is relaxing. That point is identified by another distinctive sound change, a "lub-dub." Some physiologists accept the sound as the point of diastolic pressure. This is called *fourth-phase* measurement; other physiologists wait for the complete disappearance of sound, or *fifth phase,* for measuring diastolic pressure.

During moderate to strenuous rhythmic exercise such as jogging, systolic pressure will increase while diastolic pressure remains approximately unchanged or may even decrease. In static or dynamic exercise against heavy resistance, such as weight lifting, both systolic and diastolic pressure tend to increase. The blood pressure increases much more relative to heart rate than in rhythmic exercise.

Q: *What happens when exercise causes "pooling" in the legs?*

A: During rest the blood flow through arteries and capillaries in the legs is restricted by smooth muscles in the arterial walls, which contract to hold the arteries closed and prevent excess blood from collecting by gravity in the lower extremities. This peripheral resistance to blood flow is called *vasoconstriction.* When we exercise and faster blood flow is needed, the smooth muscles relax in response to chemical changes in surrounding fluids, a process called *vasodilation.*

Vasodilation continues for some time, allowing blood to flow freely into the lower limbs. The potential accumulation of blood is nicely balanced by a massaging action of the muscles on the veins. These contain small valves that permit blood flow only toward the heart, so when muscles contract and compress the veins the blood cannot move backward or downward into the capillaries and arteries of the limbs.

However, if we suddenly stop an exercise, the free flow into the limbs continues although the venous massaging action has stopped. Blood may accumulate or "pool" in the arterioles until normal vasoconstriction once more restrains it. Sometimes the amount pooled is so great as to prevent enough blood returning to the heart to maintain an effective pumping pressure. The brain and heart may be momentarily deprived of oxygen; the person may have a fainting spell.

Blood pooling may even induce a heart attack with certain kinds of coronary disease. This possibility is the physiological rationale for "cooling off" after a period of exercise. The best way to prevent pooling of blood in the limbs is to maintain massaging action of the muscles against the veins. Do not stop suddenly after intensive jogging, for example, but instead gradually slow the pace to a walk and continue in motion for a lap or two. That way the blood vessels can gradually reestablish vasoconstriction.

Q: *What is the* Valsalva effect?

A: Named after an 18th-century anatomist, Antonio Valsalva, the effect is dizziness or fainting from holding the breath during exercise against heavy resistance.

The increased pressure in the chest cavity is transmitted to the large veins that return blood to the heart. The blood already in the veins is forced into the heart, which immediately pumps it out, with a sudden increase in blood pressure and in pulse rate. Continued pressure in the chest from continued effort prevents more blood from returning to the heart. With very little blood to pump, the blood flow and pressure suddenly decrease again, starving the brain with resultant dizziness or fainting.

During such exercises, controlled breathing in and out will periodically relieve the pressure buildup within the chest cavity, allowing blood to return to the heart and thence into normal circulation without the Valsalva effect.

Breathing and the Lungs

Q: *What is* aerobic power *and what are* aerobics?

A: Aerobics is a term popularized by Dr. Kenneth H. Cooper of the U.S. Air Force. By his own definition it refers to "a variety of exercises that stimulate heart and lung activity [typically including] running, swimming, cycling, and jogging." In biology the term "aerobic" means "living or acting only in the presence of oxygen."

The main objective of an aerobic exercise program is to increase the maximum amount of oxygen that the body can process within a given time—the maximum that can be transported from the lungs to muscular and other tissues. This amount is called a person's maximum oxygen intake, aerobic capacity, or aerobic power.

Q: *How is aerobic power used as a test of physical fitness?*

A: The amount of oxygen that can be delivered to the tissue is dependent upon a chain of physiological events. These are:

- *Ventilation,* the movement of air in and out of the lungs;
- *Diffusion,* the transfer of oxygen from the lungs to the blood;
- *Transport,* the ability of the blood to pick up oxygen,

which depends in turn on the amount of hemoglobin that the blood contains;

• *Pumping* of blood by the heart;

• *Delivery* of blood to the muscles via the arteries, arterioles, and capillaries, the efficiency of which depends upon the vascular condition; and

• *Chemical* reaction, which determines the ability of cells to use oxygen transported by the blood. This ability depends on microscopic structures called mitochondria within the cells and of certain enzymes which must be present if the chemical reactions which use oxygen are to take place. Energy is utilized by oxidizing or combining food elements with oxygen.

Like any chain, the oxygen intake chain is only as strong as its weakest link. If there is a deficiency in any function such as the amount of blood hemoglobin, the pumping ability of the heart, or distribution of blood by the arteries, a person's aerobic power will be reduced.

Training through exercise improves many of these functions. Improved heart action, improved muscle capillarization, and an increase in cell mitochondria and enzymes are commonly accepted training effects. It is not unusual to achieve improvement in aerobic power ranging from 15 to 20 percent with endurance type training programs such as those conducted by YMCA's.

A measure of maximum oxygen intake gives information about a person's work tolerance before beginning an exercise program. Later it shows up any functional improvement due to exercise. It does not diagnose pathological conditions or take the place of a medical examination. It should be combined with tests of body composition, muscular endurance, and strength to form a complete picture of a person's physical fitness status.

Note: Some people have a naturally high maximum oxygen intake, apparently due to heredity. They may do well on a physical fitness test even though not in training at the time, and would be expected to improve even more with physical conditioning. Many find success in competitive endurance activities, such as long-distance running.

Q: *What aerobic tests are used in physical fitness?*

A: The direct measurement of maximum oxygen intake is not practical except in a laboratory setting. Other tests (described in this book) are used to estimate aerobic power indirectly, along with a number of tests of respiratory functioning, as follows:

• *Vital capacity* (VC) is the maximum amount of air that a person can breathe out after taking the deepest possible breath—a basic but not definitive measure. Obviously, it takes a certain lung volume to provide an adequate amount of air and oxygen during exercise. Some studies have shown an increase in VC with training but others have not. Swimming seems to make the most improvement in VC while jogging has very little effect.

• *Time-forced vital capacity* (FVC) is similar to the VC test, but the breathing-out phase is forced to completion as rapidly as possible. It indicates the contractile strength of the expiratory muscles. Not uncommonly, FVC improves with training.

• *Forced expiratory volume in one second* (FEV$_1$) is the volume of air expired during the first second of the FVC test. Like the latter, it indicates strength of the lung muscles and may improve with training.

• *Percent of forced vital capacity expired in one second* (divide FEV$_1$ by FVC). As a rule of thumb, more than 80 percent of FVC should be breathed out in the first second. Lower values suggest lack of thoracic mobility and ineffective removal of air from the lungs. Low results in this measure are characteristic of asthmatics.

Q: *What is the relation of lung function to performance?*

A: As the intensity of exercise increases (for example, by running faster) the body's demand for air and oxygen increases. Pulmonary minute volume (PMV) is the volume of air in liters moved through the lungs per minute. There is a very close relationship between PMV and the amount of oxygen used by the body. The *maximum* ventilation level rises with training.

An untrained, middle-aged man may be able to ventilate only 40 to 80 liters of air per minute. During hard exercise, a normal male college student will ventilate about 120 liters per minute. A champion distance runner may be able to breathe over 200 liters per minute for brief periods of time— as when in support of his closing "kick."

Q: *How should one breathe while jogging?*

A: Breathing is an automatically controlled mechanism

of the body; the less you interfere with it the better. Let the body adjust as it will.

When very poorly conditioned adults first begin an exercise program they may become "winded" easily, but this is a sign of overall poor response to exercise and not a sign of need to learn how to breathe. As physical condition improves, the body will adjust better to exercise and the respiratory function will improve with it.

Q: *Do breathing exercises help?*

A: Breathing exercises are of specific benefit to persons suffering from chronic respiratory conditions such as emphysema or asthma. In others, deep breathing and diaphragm exercises promote relaxation, which may be beneficial. Whether such exercises actually improve one's ability to handle physical exertion is highly questionable. In fact, it is advisable to avoid long periods of holding the breath, especially after strenuous exercise.

Exercise and Weight Control

Q: *Is it worthwhile to consider exercise as a factor in reducing weight?*

A: This question arises because relatively few calories are expended during exercise, as compared to the reduction in calories possible through dieting. (See table, page 41.) Usually, however, it is best to reduce weight both by controlling food intake and by exercising, which has a number of important advantages.

Weight gain or loss generally follows the laws of thermodynamics. A positive energy balance (calorie intake greater than calorie expenditure) results in weight gain; the opposite results in a negative energy balance and weight loss. One pound of fat is equal to about 3,500 calories. Exercise programs such as those described in this book will expend from 400 to 500 calories per workout. The negative balance is *cumulative;* exercise at this rate is equivalent to a pound of fat lost for every seven to nine workouts.

It is true that eating a rich dessert once each day can easily cancel the calorie loss from exercise, resulting in an equivalent positive caloric balance and no weight change. But it should be remembered that exercise affects more than the body weight. Improvements in the cardiovascular, respiratory, and muscular systems are not gained by dieting alone.

Q: *Is it true, as some people claim, that exercise leads to a heightened appetite for food and thereby makes losing weight more difficult?*

A: This frequent question could be answered, "Yes and no." Yes, because authorities agree that appetite is related closely to energy expenditure over a wide range of exercise intensities; an active person does tend to eat more. No, because obesity is closely associated with physical lethargy. When a person exercises infrequently, the regulatory mechanism controlling appetite does not operate as effectively or precisely as in an active person. The appetite of an inactive person often is set for an energy supply *greater* than the need. (See Chapter 4.)

Professor Per-Olof Astrand, the Swedish expert on exercise physiology, says: "Those who are physically inactive must watch their diet very carefully and select food items rich in essential nutrients. For the physically active individual the choice of food is less important and critical . . . [we] can eat what we like!"

Q: *Can exercise "change fat to muscle"?*

A: Technically, no, but in practice, yes. When an untrained person participates in exercise there is a tendency to lose fat while increasing the amount of muscle tissue in the body composition. These are separate physiological events occurring at the same time, but with the practical effect of "changing" fat to muscle.

Q: *What is the effect of exercise on blood lipids (cholesterol, triglycerides, fats)?*

A: Intense exercise (300 to 500 calories in less than an hour) has been shown to reduce the lipids in blood serum. A definite decrease in cholesterol occurs when there is a loss of weight at the same time. Dr. Warren Guild of Harvard Medical School, a specialist in sports medicine, states that a number of exercise benefits which were once "largely hunches" have now been proved by laboratory analysis, among them: "Exercise converts fatty tissue to beneficial muscle tissue. Exercise can burn up fatty tissue. And exercise has been proven to reduce blood cholesterol levels."

Heat, Cold, and Soreness

Q: *Should special precautions be taken when exercising in the heat?*

A: Yes. First, one should wear as little clothing as possible. Second, it is necessary to replace salt lost through sweating. Most people can adequately adjust the salt intake by adding more to their food. For extreme situations of prolonged perspiration, salt tablets are available.

Give your body time to adapt to the heat. Do not exercise too strenuously during the first warm days of the season and do not wear rubber or plastic clothing to induce excessive sweating. Being physically fit helps one to tolerate heat, but is not a substitute for heat adaptation.

The only way to increase heat tolerance is to exercise regularly on warm days—and even then it is important to be cautious. When heat and humidity are high, either cut back on exercise, do more swimming than other types of activity, or do not exercise at all.

Q: *What scientific standard can be used to judge the amount of exercise tolerable in the heat?*

A: The temperature-humidity index (THI) provides the best means of evaluating heat-stress danger. The daily THI is reported for *outdoor* conditions by local weather bureaus, with a reading of 70° or above considered the "discomfort zone." To measure the THI for *indoor* activity requires the use of "wet bulb" and "dry bulb" thermometers. It is computed by the following formula and table (from D. Minard, U.S. Marine Corps):

THI = 0.67 × wet bulb temperature + 0.3 × dry bulb temperature.

Below 70	No danger.
70.1–72.5	No sweatsuits; overweight persons should reduce activity.
72.6–75.0	Reduce distance and speed of running; the overweight should limit themselves to easy calisthenics and slow jogging.
75.1–77.5	Very slow jogging and light calisthenics only; be alert for heat distress signs.
77.6–80.0	Light calisthenics, only a few laps of easy jogging. Swimming preferred.
Over 80	No gym workout—swimming pool only.

Q: *What about sauna baths, steam baths, rubberized gym clothing and other devices to "melt the fat away"?*

A: The answer involves an understanding of dehydration (water loss). A loss of body weight may be either temporary or reasonably permanent. Water is heavy (1.05 pounds per pint); therefore water lost through dehydration, whether by sweating or prolonged thirst, will be quickly reflected in loss of body weight. This "instant reducing," however, is only apparent.

Since dehydration upsets the body's water balance and thereby its chemical balance, a dehydrated individual will restore the water as soon as he can by drinking and eating. Thus any apparently lost weight will be put right back on.

Sauna and steam baths promote sweating and a water loss that looks good on the scale. But because this is dehydration, the body will conserve water during the next few hours and soon regain the lost weight. Football players on a warm day may lose five to seven pounds in perspiration during a game— but gain it back the same evening. (They may imbibe a soft drink especially concocted to restore body minerals along with the water.)

Physicians have expressed growing concern that sauna and steam bathing may be detrimental to health. Heat stress is not well tolerated by most middle-aged people. The danger of heat exhaustion is increased if an individual enters the hot bath after exercise, when the body is trying to dissipate heat and lower its temperature.

The same rationale applies to rubberized or other types of non-porous sweat suit. The material encloses the body in a hot environment that causes sweating during exercise and thereby the same sort of dehydration and temporary weight loss as a steam bath.

Sauna belts, hot pants, and other "reducing" devices made of non-porous materials retain heat in a particular area of the body, thereby promoting localized sweating. There is no evidence that this will contribute to fat reduction. A Federal Trade Commission ruling has restricted advertising claims to that effect.

Q: *What about spot reducing by massage or with vibrators?*

A: The energy cost of lying on a vibrating bench or chair or leaning into a massaging belt is extremely low

78

(0.002 calories per minute). Therefore, you can anticipate no reduction in fat as a result of the exercise done. The machine is getting all the "exercise" and consuming all the energy in the form of kilowatts.

These devices are not effective in "breaking up" fat deposits or altering the body composition in any other way. Much the same is true of hand massage; it's the masseur who gets the workout and most of the benefits. Some individuals find these techniques relaxing. A reduction of tension, temporary as it may be, is not uncommon. But there is no evidence that spot reducing is effective for the purpose of losing weight.

Q: *Should special precautions be taken when exercising in the cold?*

A: Yes. Do not exercise when you are forced to inhale deeply an excessive amount of ice-cold air. Sudden cooling of the lower neck and chest can trigger a reflex causing vasoconstriction in the heart. Its oxygen supply is reduced, leading to the onset of certain kinds of heart attacks.

When exercising in the cold, whether running, skiing, or shoveling snow, middle-aged persons should warm up adequately by working into the exercise gradually. It may be desirable to warm up indoors in some instances.

When shoveling snow, it is better to lift small loads often, even if it takes longer. Lifting a large, heavy scoop full of wet snow is no different in its physiological effects from doing heavy resistance work (such as weight lifting) in the gymnasium. Generally the person who is physically fit and accustomed to strenuous activity does not have to be as concerned as the sedentary, unfit person. In any case, the wise snow shoveler will keep a small scoop handy to avoid the temptation to lift heavy loads of snow and "get the job over with."

Q: *What causes muscle soreness in people just beginning an exercise program?*

A: Two types of pain may result from the exertion. One is pain during and immediately after exercise, which is probably due to waste products formed during exertion and left in the fluids surrounding the cells. It is temporary and should not be a deterrent to continue exercising. It can occur when trying a new exercise or when increasing the exercise intensity.

The second type is more serious, coming as a localized, delayed soreness in twenty-four to forty-eight hours after exercise. Whether it is due to small muscle tears or small localized muscle contractions is not known, but it can become chronic and will not be helped by further exercise. Chronic soreness requires medical evaluation.

Q: *Can muscle soreness be prevented?*

A: Usually, yes. A conservative approach to exercise is the key, especially a thorough warm-up. Increase the work load only gradually during exercise, and progress slowly from one workout to the next. Stay within your own tolerance level. Don't overdo a given exercise, and taper off at the end of a workout by gradually decreasing the exercise intensity. Avoid bouncing and stretching exercises that force the joints to the limits of their range of motion. However, static stretching (while standing, sitting, or reclining) has been found effective in both preventing and relieving muscle soreness.

Q: *What is the best time of day to exercise?*

A: Any convenient time is fine, with only one minor exception. Let at least one hour elapse after a heavy meal before exercising too strenuously. Far more important than the time of day is *regularity*: a person should exercise on a regular schedule two or three times each week.

Q: *What's the significance of lactic acid in exercise?*

A: Lactic acid, $C_3H_6O_3$, is formed when the body is not meeting all the demands of its cells for oxygen. For a short time the lactic acid enables the body to keep providing energy for physical activity despite the shortage of oxygen—for example, for an extra burst of speed in a race. But when lactic acid accumulates in a muscle or throughout the body, it interferes with muscular contraction and brings on fatigue. A trained person can utilize a greater percentage of his aerobic power than an untrained person before lactic acid accumulates in troublesome quantity.

Q: *How much exercise can a sedentary man tolerate?*

A: Almost anyone can start exercising at any time, but the nature of the activity to be chosen depends on a number of important factors: the individual's age, his health, whether he smokes, how inactive he has been, and for how long. For example:

A 30-year-old man who has been sedentary for ten years, does not smoke, is within normal weight limits, and is free of disease can probably handle any exercise program as long as he starts out slowly, exercises regularly, and progresses steadily. But, a 55-year-old man who has been sedentary for thirty-five years, smokes two packs of cigarettes a day, is overweight, has some history of high blood pressure, high cholesterol, and diabetes should probably undertake only a severely limited program, mostly walking and rhythmic flexibility exercises.

The limiting factors are determined by medical examination and by physical fitness testing (Chapter 7). Common sense is the guideline. One can always advance, start at a safe, low intensity of exercise, make progress cautiously, and let individual response dictate the nature of the workouts.

Girls and Women

Q: *Are training effects in women different from the training effects in men?*

A: As a humorist has said, "You can't argue with biology." There are physical differences between men and women reflected in the rate at which they respond to training, and these should be recognized. However, if the objective of exercising is increased stamina and endurance, the effects of training are eventually the same and women profit in the same way as men.

Q: *Will exercise produce heavy muscles and "defeminize" the person?*

A: Research suggests that properly designed exercise programs improve rather than hinder femininity. There certainly is nothing unattractive about champion women tennis players, swimmers, gymnasts, ballerinas, etc. Any tendency that a few women might have toward developing unwanted muscle definition can be forestalled by avoiding heavy resistance exercises, such as weight lifting. Most women (like most men) should emphasize rhythmic, endurance-type activities.

Q: *Should a woman exercise during the menstrual period?*

A: During the first two days of the menstrual period, medical opinion favors refraining from strenuous activity or intense competition. The ability to tolerate exercise varies in different women, and after the first two days each should proceed according to her own judgment. Some women athletes have won Olympic medals while menstruating.

Q: *Can exercise relieve dysmenorrhea?*

A: Dysmenorrhea (painful menstruation) is often due to inadequate abdominal strength. It is not desirable during the menstrual period for susceptible women to participate in any activity that increases abdominal pressure on the pelvic floor. That includes heavy lifting and hard landings on the feet. At other times of the month, suitable exercises for abdominal strengthening and lateral trunk flexibility should help correct the condition.

Q: *Can women engage in jogging and other endurance exercises?*

A: There is no reason why they can't, but their standards of performance cannot be the same as for the male. Women tend to have a poorer oxygen delivery system than men. On the average, they have less blood hemoglobin (the oxygen carrying substance), smaller volume of blood, a lower stroke volume of the heart, and less muscle capillarization—in sum, a lower oxygen intake per kilogram of body weight.

All of these explain why females cannot compete in athletics or strenuous work on the same plane as males. Within feminine parameters of performance, however, women can participate in endurance activities and gain great benefits from them.

Basic Principles for Body Conditioning

In this discussion of exercise physiology, exercise has not been conceived as an indiscriminate activity, but as a planned, regular, and scientifically programmed course of action. In setting up such a program, five principles are followed, whether by the physical director of a YMCA or by an individual establishing his own schedule and objectives.

1. Overload Principle

In order to accomplish body conditioning and physical fitness improvement, the body must do more work than it normally does.

For some people the amount of overload necessary is surprisingly small; fast walking may be all they need to produce measurable results in body condition. In an exercise program, overload is accomplished in two principal ways: (1) by increasing the total work a person does (e.g., run further), which is emphasized during early exercise sessions, and (2) increasing the work rate (e.g., run faster), which is applied as the participant becomes better conditioned.

II. Progression Principle

If physical condition is to be improved, a person must be repeatedly exposed to new, higher levels of overload.

As one continually handles a given work load, the body makes physiological adjustments and becomes adapted to it. Hence this level of exercise no longer is an "overload" and it is necessary to progress to a new overload, that is, to undertake more difficult or demanding exercise routines as condition improves.

Not all individuals improve at the same rate; hence, competitive attitudes are discouraged in group conditioning sessions. Through a series of overloads, each person will reach a level of physical fitness that he considers high enough *for him*. At that point he probably should look for a combination of exercises and sports that will hold his interest and keep him active.

III. Use-Disuse Principle

Use promotes function, disuse promotes deterioration, whether of the body as a whole or of its parts taken separately.

For this reason, a good exercise program will be planned to include all components of physical fitness (endurance, flexibility, strength) and all of the muscles. The use-disuse principle also makes necessary a minimum frequency of exercise. Three sessions a week of forty-five minutes to an hour are recommended. Two sessions a week are generally considered the absolute minimum to achieve any consistent training effect.

IV. Specificity Principle

Specific improvements in physical fitness are produced by specific kinds of training. The body responds directly to the demands placed upon it, and the effects are not interchangeable.

Thus, aerobic exercises develop cardiorespiratory endurance, stretching exercises develop flexibility, and resistance exercises develop strength. As stated above, a good exercise program should include all components of fitness; furthermore, rates of progress should be established for improvement of each specific quality desired.

V. Individual Differences Principle

Each person responds to a training program in his own way at his own rate.

Factors related to the individual rate of response are a person's age, body type, degree of obesity, habits of rest and sleep, nutrition, injury and disease, and motivation. Some people should walk while others run; some may do bent-knee sit-ups while others are only able to lift their shoulders from the floor. A good program allows for this, and avoids competition between participants.

The remaining chapters in this book will help you determine your own level of tolerance for exercise and a suitable rate of progress toward body conditioning.

Chapter 7

HOW DO YOU MEASURE UP?

A modern body conditioning program such as those developed by the YMCA attaches great significance to certain physical tests of each individual. In the past, people often undertook exercise or sports on a personal preference, "hunch," or hit-or-miss basis, sometimes with inconclusive or even negative results. Through scientific evaluation, we can find out how we measure up physically and set up our conditioning programs accordingly.

These fitness measures are commonly made before, during, and after exercising. The preliminary tests determine whether you will benefit by exercise, and help to set a level of intensity commensurate with your ability to tolerate exertion. Testing is especially important as a precaution for middle-aged or out-of-shape individuals. Later tests made in the course of pursuing a program objective show what the exercise is doing for you, supplying a scientific measure of progress. Postexercise tests complete the before-and-after picture.

The last may be the most gratifying to one's self-esteem, but the first or preliminary tests are the most vital to your health. They fall into two categories: medical evaluation made by a physician and physical fitness evaluation made by the director of your fitness program or even by yourself. One such evaluation test has already been described in this book, the measurement of body composition to determine percent of fat and ideal body weight (Chapter 5).

Medical Evaluation

A thorough physical examination by a doctor is a *must* on your road to physical fitness. The older you are, the more essential this becomes. Dr. Kenneth Cooper in his aerobics program establishes the following age guidelines or exam requirements:

Up to age 30: A complete physical examination *within the past year.* You can start exercising now and choose any type of activity that interests you, if the doctor found nothing wrong.

Up to age 40: A complete physical examination *within the past three months,* including an electrocardiogram (EKG) of the usual type, that is, recorded with the patient at rest. The doctor should also take down a full record of your past health history.

Up to age 60: Same as the foregoing with one addition; a second EKG should be taken *while exercising.* This is now regarded as the really meaningful measure, even if you have to search for a YMCA with a physical fitness testing center or for a doctor equipped to give an "exercise EKG." Your pulse rate from the stress imposed during this test should approach the level likely to be reached during the kind of fitness activity chosen (e.g., in running, swimming, tennis, etc.). The table on page 87 shows target heart rates for an exercise EKG at various ages.

Age 60 and over: Same as the preceding except that the complete physical exam, including electrocardiograms both at rest and during exercise and the lifetime health history, should be performed *immediately before* starting the exercise program.

Exercise and Age

Even in the absence of actual medical problems, the aging process gradually lowers the efficiency of the heart, arteries, and lungs and thereby the permissible limits of physical activity for an individual. Every athlete knows this. A ballplayer or boxer considers himself "old" at 30, "over the hill" at 35, and ready for a retirement pension at 40. Most of us are not athletes and we resist thinking of ourselves as old until the postman starts delivering Social Security checks—if even then! Nevertheless the years progressively lower one's ability to "take it," as shown by the following table.

These are target heart rates used by physicians during EKG stress testing, primarily to determine the presence or absence of heart disease, but also useful in planning the intensity of an exercise program. Note that the target rate decreases about one heart beat per year of age.

Age (Years)	Target Heart Rate* (Maximum beats per minute)
Under 30	175
30–34	170
35–39	165
40–44	160
45–49	155
50–54	150
55–59	145
60–64	140
65 and up	135

*(From *The New Aerobics* by Kenneth H. Cooper, M.D. Copyright © 1970 by Kenneth H. Cooper. Reprinted by permission of the publisher, M. Evans and Company, Inc., New York, N.Y. 10017.)

As signaled by the heart rate—a measure of how far the heart can be safely pushed—the years divide us into four approximate exercise categories and suggest the kinds of activity that will suit us best. Despite some outstanding individual exceptions, most people will be well advised to go along with their natural limitations. As the margarine ad says, "It's not *nice* to fool Mother Nature!"

Up to age 30: Unless the physical examination discloses some significant handicap or provokes a warning from the doctor, you can do any kind of exercise you want—run, jog, swim, cycle, play handball, anything you enjoy that regularly exerts your muscles.

From 30 to 50: If in condition, you're almost as good as ever but the fine edge is wearing off. You can have your choice of exercise routines or sports, but before indulging in anything really strenuous (e.g., squash, handball), take the precaution of getting your doctor's O.K.

From 50 to 60: A difficulty here is not just the natural aging imposed on the body by the calendar but the contrariness of human nature. A well-conditioned person of middle age can do almost as well as younger men. He can even beat younger men who are in flabby shape. But often a person who *starts* a body conditioning program after age 50 is trying to make up overnight for twenty or thirty years of neglect.

That's why the health history and physical activity profile (page 89) are important parts of the preliminary tests.

Sedentary people in their fifties are best advised to start with a walking program to achieve basic body conditioning. Don't be in a hurry, but don't be easily discouraged, either. You can still condition a middle-aged body, but it may take longer. Only when you again measure up to physical fitness standards should you consider jogging, running, or competitive sports, and then only after getting a second checkup from your doctor. You'll be safer sticking to less arduous action such as walking, swimming, cycling, or even golf (without that electric cart).

Over age 60: Walking, swimming, and cycling do the most good for most sedentary people in the sixties, who should avoid jogging, running, and vigorous competitive sports. But a senior citizen who has kept himself physically fit over the years can safely participate in jogging or running well into and even beyond the sixties. Remember the late King of Sweden who continued to play a good game of tennis at the age of 90? People in their eighties climb Mt. Washington in New Hampshire. However, if over 60, engage in strenuous sports only after basic conditioning, and then only with medical approval.

Again let us say that this limitation need not discourage exercise for body improvement. A walking program faithfully followed can eventually produce a fit body. In appearance, in vigor, in mental alertness, *just walking* every day can take 15 years off your age.

Answer the questions in the Physical Activity Profile (page 89), which will give an indication of how you measure up physically in your daily way of life. What you do every day can make an enormous difference. A famous study in England years ago set the pattern for modern cardiovascular research by comparing heart disease rates among bus drivers and bus conductors. The bus drivers sat at the wheel all day; the conductors hopped up- and downstairs in the double-decked vehicles. They had a much lower incidence of heart attacks than the unexercised drivers.

Medical Exam Criteria

As mentioned earlier, you might have to shop around a bit for a doctor equipped for and interested in performing

PHYSICAL ACTIVITY PROFILE

NAME_____ DATE_____

Please answer the following questions about your job- and non-job-related phsyical activity.

(1) WHAT TYPE OF WORK DO YOU DO? (For example, store manager, teacher, lawyer)

_____

(2) IN WHAT KIND OF BUSINESS OR INDUSTRY DO YOU WORK? (For example, electronics, manufacturing, insurance company, food store)

_____

(3) ON THE AVERAGE DURING THE PAST YEAR, HOW MANY HOURS PER DAY HAVE YOU SPENT PERFORMING THE FOLLOWING ACTIVITIES *WHILE AT WORK?* (Include time spent going to and from work)

Activity	Hours per day
Sitting, e.g. typing, writing, reading, etc. (Not including driving)	_____
Driving auto, truck, bus, or other equipment	_____
Standing	_____
Walking	_____
Light physical labor, e.g., work at lathe, or other equipment	_____
Moderate physical labor, e.g., using tools such as hammer, wrenches, etc.	_____
Heavy physical labor, e.g., lifting or carrying heavy objects, digging, chopping wood	_____
Other. Specify_____	_____

(4) HOW WOULD YOU RATE THE AMOUNT OF PHYSICAL ACTIVITY YOU PERFORM WHILE AT WORK?

very little	little	moderate	active	very active
/	/	/	/	/

(5) HOW WOULD YOU RATE THE AMOUNT OF PHYSICAL ACTIVITY YOU PERFORM DURING YOUR LEISURE TIME?

___/_____/_____/_____/_____/___

very little   little   moderate   active   very active

(6) ARE YOU PRESENTLY PERFORMING ANY STANDARD "PHYSICAL FITNESS" PROGRAM? (For example, Aerobics, Canadian 5BX)
YES_____ NO_____
If yes, which one?_____

(7) HOW *PHYSICALLY FIT* DO YOU FEEL AT THE PRESENT?

___/_____/_____/_____/_____/___

unfit   below average   average   above average   very fit

(8) PROVIDING THE EQUIPMENT AND FACILITIES WERE AVAILABLE, IN WHICH PHYSICAL ACTIVITIES WOULD YOU BE INTERESTED IN LEARNING AND PARTICIPATING? PLEASE CHECK OR LIST ACTIVITIES.

Hiking _____	Tennis _____	Calisthenics _____
Jogging _____	Handball _____	Weight train-
Bicycling _____	Volleyball _____	ing _____
Swimming _____	Badminton _____	Golf _____
		Supervised conditioning program _____

Other (Specify)

_____
_____
_____
_____

(9) DO YOU HAVE ANY EXERCISE EQUIPMENT OR DEVICE AT HOME?
YES_____ NO_____
If yes, please specify _____

the kind of physical examination recommended for exercise planning, especially an exercise EKG. This is not a criticism of the profession but a matter of emphasis in training. Until ten or fifteen years ago most medical schools emphasized chemotherapy (prescription of medicines) to virtually the complete neglect of physiotherapy, which is concerned with the nutritional and exercise factors in health. Today physical medicine, like space medicine, is an emerging specialty.

On page 92 is an outline for a model physical examination and health history. You can answer many of the questions yourself. The YMCA lists the following items as (a) required and essential or (b) optional and desirable in preliminary medical examinations of new members.

a. Required Items
    Complete medical history
    Physical examination including auscultation
        (listening with stethoscope), heart
        rate, and blood pressure
    Electrocardiogram at rest
    Electrocardiogram during exercise
        (stress test)

b. Optional Items
    Blood analysis including lipid profile
        (cholesterol, triglycerides,
        lipoprotein in blood serum), glucose,
        uric acid, complete blood count (CBC),
        hemoglobin, hematocrit
    Urinalysis, including glucose and protein
    Chest X-ray
    Lung function, including forced expiratory
        volume (FEV) in 1 second and 3 seconds
    Coronary risk profile (page 98)
    Physical Activity Profile (page 89)

Taking Your Pulse

Since the heart rate is a key signal in much physical fitness testing, you should know how to take your own pulse accurately. It can be done even while running or jogging, as a check on the progress of your improvement as well as a precaution against overexertion.

You may have tried to take your pulse at the wrist with inconclusive results. Your own heart beat does not come

HISTORY AND PHYSICAL EXAMINATION

NAME _____

DATE _____ AGE _____

1. *GENERAL MEDICAL HISTORY*   *circle one*

Any medical complaints? _____	YES NO
Any major illnesses in the past? (Give dates.)	YES NO
Any hospitalization?	YES NO

Smoke now? _____ Packages per day __	YES NO
Smoked in past? _____ Packages per day __	YES NO
Weight gain in past ten years _____ lbs. _____	YES NO
Weight at age 20_____ 30_____ 40_____ 50_____	
Diabetes? _____	YES NO
Family history of diabetes? Who? _____	YES NO
Family history of heart disease? _____	YES NO
Who? _____	
Family history of high blood pressure? _____	YES NO
Who? _____	
Family history of muscular illness? _____	YES NO
Who? _____	

2. *CARDIORESPIRATORY HISTORY*

Any heart disease now?	YES NO	Daily coughing?	YES NO
Any heart disease in past?	YES NO	Cough produces sputum?	YES NO
Heart murmurs?	YES NO	High blood pressure?	YES NO
Occasional chest pains?	YES NO	Shortness of breath at rest?	YES NO
Chest pains on exertion?	YES NO	Shortness of breath supine?	YES NO
Chest pressure on exertion?	YES NO	Shortness of breath after two flights	
Fainting?	YES NO	of stairs?	YES NO

3. *MUSCULAR HISTORY*

Any muscle injuries or illnesses now? YES NO

Muscular illness now? YES NO

Any muscle injuries or illness in past? YES NO

Muscle pain at rest? YES NO

Muscular weakness now? YES NO

Muscle pains at exertion? YES NO

4. BONE-JOINT HISTORY

Any bone or joint (including spine) injuries or illness now? YES NO

Ever had painful joints? YES NO

Flat feet? YES NO

Any bones or joint (including spine) injuries or illness in past? YES NO

Athletics in past? YES NO
Specify _____
_____
_____

Ever had swollen joints? YES NO

_____
_____

5. LABORATORY EXAMINATION

Height _____ Weight _____ Waist girth _____

Fat thickness triceps _____ Scapula _____

Vital capacity _____

Forced expiratory volume (1 sec.) _____

ECG rate _____ Rhythm _____

Axis _____

Interpretation _____

BLOOD hematocrit _____ Hemoglobin _____

White cell count _____

Cholesterol (fasting) _____

Blood sugar (2 hr. after meal) _____

URINALYSIS Special gravity _____

Protein _____

Sugar _____

CHEST X-RAY Interpretation _____

PHYSICAL EXAMINATION

Thyroid abnormal? YES NO

Gallops, abnormal heart sounds? YES NO

Chest auscultation abnormal? YES NO

Any joints abnormal? YES NO

Heart size abnormal? YES NO

Abnormal masses? YES NO

Murmurs present? YES NO

Hernias? YES NO

Peripheral pulses absent? YES NO

93

SUMMARY IMPRESSION OF PHYSICIAN

1. Comments on any history or physical finding (especially "yes" answers)

_____

_____

_____

Diagnoses _____

_____

2. *RECOMMENDATIONS:*
    (1) There is *no contraindication* to participation in a moderately vigorous general exercise program.

OR
    (2) Because of the above diagnosis, participation in a moderately vigorous general exercise program *may be advisable* and further examination or consultation is necessary, namely: _____

_____

OR
    (3) Because of the above diagnosis, participation in a moderately vigorous general exercise program is inadvisable.

RELEASE
    I hereby release the above information to the Exercise Program Director.

        SIGNED: _____

through strongly enough at that point, although you could readily feel another person's wrist pulse. Instead, feel for your own pulse in the neck artery, below the jawbone at approximately the neckline of a shirt collar. Press firmly with the index and second fingers of either hand while keeping your eye on the sweephand of a wristwatch.

Doctors and nurses count the pulse for ten seconds and multiply by six to get the heart rate in beats per minute. Or you can count for fifteen seconds and multiply by four, or for twenty seconds times three, etc. The longer the period of counting the pulse at rest, the more accurate the result is apt to be.

Using a stopwatch, an even more accurate pulse results from measuring the time it takes to count thirty beats. Count to the nearest tenth of a second. To get the heart rate, divide the stopwatch time into 1,800 as shown by this formula:

$$\text{Heart rate/min.} = \frac{60 \text{ sec.}}{\text{Time in sec.}} \times 30 \text{ beats} = \frac{1800}{\text{Time in sec.}}$$

The conversion table on page 96 does the arithmetic for you.

The pulse or heart rate is directly related to physical endurance. It speeds up during exertion in a normal person, but speeds up too much when body condition and fitness are less than adequate. The heart also recovers from exertion more quickly in fit people than in the unfit, slowing down to the normal beat of the heart at rest within a certain number of minutes or seconds.

To measure the rate of recovery, the pulse is taken after five minutes or ten minutes of rest following exercise. These measures—maximum exercising heart beat and heart recovery rate—are then compared to norms established for people of various ages and fitness levels in laboratory experiments.

Contraindications to Exercise

Medical opinion regarding exercise is in the process of change. At one time anyone with "heart trouble" was advised to rest, take it easy, avoid exertion of any kind. Today, he is told to keep active, to exercise intelligently, to move his muscles every day. A victim of intermittent claudication, a clogging of blood vessels in the legs that causes muscular pain with walking, is told to walk, *walk*, WALK as long and as far as he can stand it. Today, exercise is recommended as a therapy for this condition rather than discouraged as a source of potential harm.

Nevertheless, there are some pathological conditions that a physician will tell you indicate that exercise is not for you. The YMCA lists these contraindications under various categories for the guidance of its physical directors. Some disorders bar *any* exercise at all, some put a *limit* on the intensity or amount of exercise permitted, and some contraindicate *unsupervised* activity (i.e., the individual can exercise but only under professional supervision).

Limiting Conditions for Exercise

General medical problems restricting *unsupervised* participation in an exercise program include:

HEART RATE CONVERSION (TIME FOR 30 BEATS TO RATE/MIN.)

22.0 SEC.	82/MIN.	17.3 SEC.	104/MIN.	12.6 SEC.	143/MIN.
21.9	82	17.2	105	12.5	144
21.8	83	17.1	105	12.4	145
21.7	83	17.0	106	12.3	146
21.6	83	16.9	107	12.2	148
21.5	84	16.8	107	12.1	149
21.4	84	16.7	108	12.0	150
21.3	85	16.6	108	11.9	151
21.2	85	16.5	109	11.8	153
21.1	85	16.4	110	11.7	154
21.0	86	16.3	110	11.6	155
20.9	86	16.2	111	11.5	157
20.8	87	16.1	112	11.4	158
20.7	87	16.0	113	11.3	159
20.6	87	15.9	113	11.2	161
20.5	88	15.8	114	11.1	162
20.4	88	15.7	115	11.0	164
20.3	89	15.6	115	10.9	165
20.2	89	15.5	116	10.8	167
20.1	90	15.4	117	10.7	168
20.0	90	15.3	118	10.6	170
19.9	90	15.2	118	10.5	171
19.8	91	15.1	119	10.4	173
19.7	91	15.0	120	10.3	175
19.6	92	14.9	121	10.2	176
19.5	92	14.8	122	10.1	178
19.4	93	14.7	122	10.0	180
19.3	93	14.6	123	9.9	182
19.2	94	14.5	124	9.8	184
19.1	94	14.4	125	9.7	186
19.0	95	14.3	126	9.6	188
18.9	95	14.2	127	9.5	189
18.8	96	14.1	128	9.4	191
18.7	96	14.0	129	9.3	194
18.6	97	13.9	129	9.2	196
18.5	97	13.8	130	9.1	198
18.4	98	13.7	131	9.0	200
18.3	98	13.6	132	8.9	202
18.2	99	13.5	133	8.8	205
18.1	99	13.4	134	8.7	207
18.0	100	13.3	135	8.6	209
17.9	101	13.2	136	8.5	212
17.8	101	13.1	137	8.4	214
17.7	102	13.0	138	8.3	217
17.6	102	12.9	140	8.2	220
17.5	103	12.8	141	8.1	222
17.4	103	12.7	142	8.0	225

- Any infectious disease during the acute or chronic stage.
- Diabetes mellitus requiring insulin injections.
- Liver disease, particularly when jaundice is present.
- Diseases involving hemorrhage, including anemia under treatment but not yet corrected, i.e., less than 10 gm./100 cc.
- History of recent or active gastrointestinal bleeding, e.g., from stomach ulcers.
- History of recent surgery, until the patient is completely ambulatory.

- Kidney disease, chronic or acute, and acidosis.
- Acute or chronic lung disease, severe pulmonary insufficiency, or both.

Cardiovascular problems that *restrict* or in certain cases *prohibit* exercise include:

- Coronary or valvular heart disease, acquired or congenital. Patients with rheumatic heart disease that has left valvular lesions should not participate in competitive sports, irrespective of symptoms.
- Any significant EKG abnormality, although by themselves the following need not restrict participation in exercise: axis deviation, intraventricular block, hypervoltage, frequent premature ventricular contractions, or old infarct pattern.
- Cardiac problems of doubtful significance; they should be studied by catheterization and angiography before exercise is permitted.
- Hypertension on an organic basis, i.e., blood pressure above 180/110 mm. Hg., unless there is no sign of target organ involvement.
- Peripheral vascular disease that produces impairment, such as intermittent claudication or venous thrombophlebitis or both—but temperate exercises such as walking may be indicated for their beneficial effects in relieving symptoms.

Certain musculoskeletal problems put a definite *limit* on exercise for obvious reasons, including:

- Fractures, dislocations, tendon or cartilage injuries affecting locomotion during the period of injury.
- Any arthritic condition requiring frequent medication.
- Functional inadequacy of muscles, bones, and joints, congenital or acquired.

Neurological conditions that *contraindicate* exercise include:

- Convulsive disorder not completely controlled by medication.
- History of intracranial bleeding within the last year.

Although not listed here, any disorder that a physician may deem *prohibitive* to stress testing or regular exercise should not be overlooked or ignored. Cardiovascular risk factors are shown in the chart on page 98.

CARDIOVASCULAR DISEASE RISK PROFILE

	DECREASING RISK			INCREASING RISK		
Age	25	35	45	55	65	75
C.V. Disease in Family	None	1 Blood Relative			2 Blood Relatives	
Cigarette Smoking	None	<10/day	10-20/day		20-30/day	>30/day
Blood Pressure						
Systolic	<120	140		160		180
Diastolic	<85	90	95	100	105	110
Obesity (% Fat)	<20%	25%	30%		35%	40%
Blood Chemistry						
Cholesterol	<220	240	260		300	350
Triglycerides	<100	200		300	400	>500
Glucose (1 hr. pp)	<100	140		160		>180
Physical Activity Habits	Active		Moderately Active			Inactive
Max. O₂ Consumption	High	Good	Average	Fair	Poor	
Resting Heart Rate	<65	75	85	>95		
Electrocardiogram						
Resting	Normal			Borderline		Abnormal
Exercise	Normal		Borderline			Abnormal
Pulmonary Function	Normal		Borderline			Abnormal
Stress and Tension	Under Control			Fair Control		Poorly Controlled
Other						

Chapter 8

BODY CONDITIONING TESTS

In the exercise physiology laboratory, aerobic power is measured directly: the maximum amount of oxygen the body can process during intense effort. A man walks or runs on a motor-driven treadmill with a meteorological balloon attached to his mouth and nose to collect the air he exhales. Analysis of the exhalations shows the amount of oxygen his body has used up for the exertion.

When the treadmill is speeded up or tilted uphill, the man may be worked close to the point of exhaustion. The amount of oxygen used at this maximum pace is his aerobic capacity or fitness index (measured in *ml./kg./min.*, milliliters of oxygen per kilogram of body weight per minute). A similar test can be made using a bicycle ergometer in place of the treadmill.

The significance of the test is the relationship between oxygen consumption and physical fitness. A person in very poor condition can transport less than 25 ml./kg./min. of oxygen in his bloodstream. A young athlete can transport more than twice as much, which means he can perform twice as much work, or the same work in half the time. Good to excellent scores at various ages are:

Under 30	42.5 to 51.5 ml./kg./min.
30–39	39.0 to 48.0 "
40–49	35.5 to 45.0 "
Over 50	34.0 to 43.0 "

Since this type of testing is impractical outside of the laboratory, charts have been computed which relate aerobic power to the heart rate alone.

Three-Minute Step Test

One stress test that requires only minimum equipment is simple enough to be self-administered. It is a variation of the Master two-step test introduced thirty years ago by the late Dr. Arthur M. Master, a New York cardiologist, and familiar to all physicians. The modern version was developed by Fred W. Kasch Ph.D. at San Diego State College and is known as the Kasch pulse recovery test.

This test can be taken by persons of all age groups and both sexes. Only the infirm or extremely unfit would find it too strenuous. However, *do not* try it without professional supervision if you already find the exertion of walking upstairs somewhat taxing. Abandon the step test at once if it brings on cardiac symptoms such as severe shortness of breath, tightness or pain in the chest, lightheadedness or dizziness, loss of muscle control, or nausea.

Basically you don't need *any* test to start walking for healthful activity.

On the day of testing, you should refrain from any physical exertion such as formal exercise. *Don't smoke.* Abstain from eating for two hours preceding the test.

You will need a sturdy bench twelve inches high for stepping up and down. Alternatively, find a stairway with risers about six inches high and step up to the second step. Have a clock handy with a sweep second hand, or a stopwatch, to measure the three-minute duration of the test and the heart rate afterward.

What you are going to do is step up to and down from the bench for three minutes at the rate of twenty-four steps per minute. Use a musician's metronome to set the exact pace at four counts per step or ninety-six counts per minute. Without a metronome, try experimenting ahead of time with the stopwatch and tapping a finger to fix the 24-per-minute pace in your mind.

The correct stepping procedure is in four counts: (1) step up with the right foot, (2) bring up the left foot, (3) step down with the right foot, (4) step down with the left foot, and repeat. Extend the legs fully when stepping up. Each step, up or down, is one count on the metronome, so that you step up and down with both feet twenty-four times each minute (96 counts).

After exactly three minutes of this, sit down on the bench

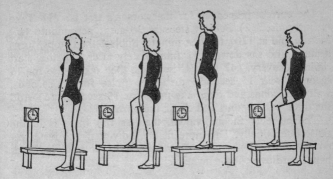

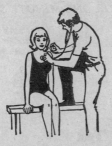

and relax, without talking. Within five seconds, take your pulse. Count the heart rate for a full minute. This is your *5-second pulse recovery,* which can then be compared to the norms for middle-aged males in the following table:

NORMS FOR 3-MINUTE STEP TEST
(HEART RATE AFTER 5 SECONDS)

Condition	Heart rate per minute
Excellent	75–80
Good	85–90
Average	95–115
Fair	120–125
Poor	130–135

One-Minute Step Test for Women

You will need the following equipment: an 18-inch-high bench, a metronome, a stopwatch, a score sheet, and a stethoscope (optional).

The correct procedure for the women's test is: (1) Take resting pulse. (2) Subject steps at 30 steps per minute (set metronome at 120) for one minute. Subject then stops, turns around, and sits down. (3) Immediately after stepping, start timing recovery. (4) Wait 15 seconds, then take pulse for 15 seconds; wait 15 seconds, then take pulse for 15 seconds; wait 15 seconds and then take pulse for 15 seconds. (5) Add the three pulse counts and check the norm table.

The more fit the individual, the less rise there is in the pulse rate initially. The more fit the individual, the faster recovery of the pulse rate. Therefore, a lower total indicates better cardiovascular efficiency.

NORMS FOR ONE-MINUTE STEP TEST

Rating	Heart rate
Excellent	66–77
Good	80–91
Average	95–109
Fair	112–123
Poor	127–137

Trunk Flexion Test

While cardiovascular endurance has been emphasized so far in these preliminary tests, and properly so, the heart is not the only common indicator of physical fitness. Lower back pain has become so prevalent a problem as to be considered by some authorities a species of epidemic. It is semi-crippling in its effects, yet almost directly related to lack of body condition. Obesity, flabby muscles, and consequent distortion of posture impose a strain on the skeletal structure that leads to pain in movement.

Specifically, lower back pain and disability among the middle-aged are related to impaired flexibility of the hip and back and reduced elasticity of the hamstring muscles. It is probable that cases of lower back pain can be improved if not cured by a carefully planned program of exercise to stretch these muscles. The degree of flexibility (or lack of it) in the skeletomuscular system therefore is a key measure of general physical fitness.

Since body flexibility is specific to each moving joint, it is difficult to measure as an overall quality. The trunk flexion test appears to give a sufficiently accurate indicator of general body flexibility. It also is specific to the lower back pain problem, whether existing or potential.

Before taking this test, a few warm-up stretching exercises (Chapter 9) are recommended. They should include bending the trunk sideways and trunk rotation. In bending laterally, one spinal muscle set contracts and the other relaxes, which makes forward trunk flexion easier. The warm-up also is a precaution against accidentally pulling a muscle with too vigorous a motion during the test.

Trunk flexion movements should be made slowly and gradually; avoid fast, jerky motions that could cause trouble. Don't try to force extreme motion against a stiff, resistant joint or taut muscles. With these caveats in mind, proceed as follows:

1. Sit on the floor with the legs extended and the heels about five inches apart.

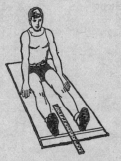

2. With a strip of adhesive tape, mark where the heels touch the floor. The heels should reach the near edge of the tape.

3. Place a yardstick on the floor between and parallel to the legs so that the 15-inch mark touches the near edge of the taped heel line.

4. Slowly reach with both hands as far forward as possible. Touch the fingertips to the yardstick and hold this position momentarily. The yardstick shows the distance reached.

5. Try this three times, recording the distance in inches each time. Do not attempt to add length by jerking forward. Your flexibility score is the best of the three trials.

Compare the result to the following norms established by the performance of adult men and women:

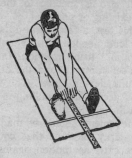

TRUNK FLEXION RATINGS

Men

Excellent	22–23 in.
Good	20–21 in.
Average	14–18 in.
Fair	12–13 in.
Poor	10–11 in.

Women

Excellent	24–27 in.
Good	21–23 in.
Average	16–20 in.
Fair	13–16 in.
Poor	0–12 in.

Muscular Strength Test

Two other important components of physical fitness are the strength and endurance of the muscles. Having superior muscular strength, a person can perform any task involving those muscles with greater ease and control. With muscular endurance, he can perform the same tasks for a longer period of time without undue fatigue.

Muscular strength for the entire body cannot be precisely measured because there are so many different muscles and muscle groups to consider. What can be measured is the strength of an individual muscle group that correlates closely with average muscle strength throughout the body.

One test commonly used by physical educators involves the hand grip. You squeeze a device that has a resistance measured in kilograms as shown on a dynamometer. Use the right hand if right-handed and vice versa. Ratings of the one-hand grip strength for men range from excellent to poor according to the device used and its calibration. Generally, 30 to 34 kilograms is poor, 66 to 70 kilograms is good.

For women, the range is 7 to 12 kilograms for poor to 35 to 40 kilograms for excellent rating.

Muscular Endurance Test

Like strength, endurance of the muscles is difficult to measure in so complicated a machine as the human body. But again, it can be estimated for exercise planning purposes by a test fairly representative of the body's overall muscular endurance. Timed sit-ups have been chosen for this purpose because they require no particular learned technique.

To take this test, you will need a partner to hold your ankles and a stopwatch or clock with sweephand to time one minute.

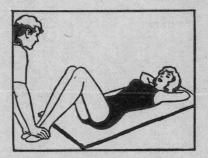

1. Lie on the floor on the back with knees bent so that the heels are about eighteen inches away from the buttocks. Your partner holds your ankles to the floor. Clasp hands behind the head.

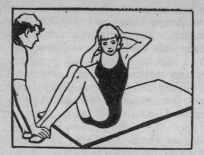

2. Do a series of sit-ups: with the right elbow touch the left knee, lie down again, then with the left elbow touch the right knee, and repeat. Each touching constitutes one sit-up and your partner maintains the count. After each sit-up return to full starting position with back to the floor. Breathe freely during the exercise; be careful not to hold the breath.

3. Do sit-ups for exactly one minute and write down the number completed. Then compare your endurance score to the following norms for adult men and women.

ONE-MINUTE SIT-UPS

Men

Excellent	35–39
Good	30–34
Average	20–29
Fair	15–19
Poor	10–14

Women

Excellent	46–54
Good	35–45
Average	22–33
Fair	12–20
Poor	2–9

Post-Exercise Testing

After your body conditioning program (including jogging) has progressed satisfactorily for several months, you might wish to look for further signs of improvement. Running to catch a bus no longer leaves you winded but that might not be a specific enough measurement for you. Body conditioning is a slow, steady—above all, *regular*—procedure, and measuring its progress realistically requires a more scientific set of facts than one's general impressions.

A *twelve-minute distance test* can supply the answers. All you have to do is to cover as great a distance as you can in twelve minutes by the clock. Run, walk, jog, stop to catch your breath—it doesn't matter, though you should push yourself a bit to do your best. Be careful not to attempt this test before you are conditioned to some degree and fully capable of handling it.

If you run or walk along a road, mark the point you reach in twelve minutes and then drive the same route in a car, measuring the distance on the car's odometer. On the running track of an athletic field or gymnasium, count the laps and multiply by the lap length, which information should be available.

It has been found that the distance covered in twelve minutes is closely related to oxygen uptake as measured in the laboratory by a treadmill or ergometer test. Therefore, if you find as a conditioning program continues that you can gradually increase the twelve-minute distance, the percent of increase statistically measures the extent of improvement in fitness. A 30 percent improvement is not uncommon in less than a year of conditioning.

Meaning of 12-Minute Tests

To get an idea of the meaning of a 12-minute distance, consider that record-breaking Olympic runners will cover a mile in less than four minutes, two miles in less than nine minutes, and three miles in less than fourteen minutes. In twelve minutes, these champions could run more than two and one half miles. For contrast, a brisk (but not forced) walking pace of four miles per hour takes you four-fifths of a mile in twelve minutes, or about sixteen city blocks.

In the 12-minute test, any distance score less than one mile indicates poor physical fitness in a male adult of any age. Anything over a mile and a half indicates good to excellent shape. For women, the standards are 5 to 10 percent lower, as in the following tables.

FITNESS RATINGS BY DISTANCE (MILES) COVERED IN 12 MINUTES*

Men

Age:	Under 30	30–39	40–49	50 & Over
Very poor	Below 1.0	Below .95	Below .85	Below .8
Poor	Up to 1.25	Up to 1.15	Up to 1.05	Up to 1.0
Average	Up to 1.5	Up to 1.4	Up to 1.3	Up to 1.25
Good	Up to 1.75	Up to 1.65	Up to 1.55	Up to 1.5
Excellent	Over 1.75	Over 1.65	Over 1.55	Over 1.5

Women

Age:	Under 30	30–39	40–49	50 & Over
Very poor	Below .95	Below .85	Below .75	Below .65
Poor	Up to 1.15	Up to 1.05	Up to .95	Up to .85
Average	Up to 1.35	Up to 1.25	Up to 1.15	Up to 1.05
Good	Up to 1.65	Up to 1.55	Up to 1.45	Up to 1.35
Excellent	Over 1.65	Over 1.55	Over 1.45	Over 1.35

*(From *The New Aerobics* by Kenneth H. Cooper, M.D. Copyright © 1970 by Kenneth H. Cooper. Reprinted by permission of the publisher, M. Evans and Company, Inc., New York, N.Y. 10017.)

The 1½-Mile Run

A 12-minute distance test is time-consuming and for that reason difficult to administer to a group of participants. As a substitute, Dr. K. H. Cooper and others have developed fitness standards related to speed (instead of distance) over a fixed course of one and one half miles. The run produces fitness rankings very similar to those of the 12-minute test. There is one important difference, however:

A 1½-mile run is a "graduate" rather than a "beginner's" test. It requires a sustained effort of large muscle groups in a strenuous task, almost an exhausting effort. *Therefore the 1½-mile run should* NOT *be attempted at all except by persons in reasonably good physical condition,* and certainly not by the grossly overweight or by those with cardiac risk symptoms (page 98). Such people can scarcely run a city block, much less thirty blocks (a mile and a half).

The YMCA recommends taking this test only after at least ten weeks of fitness training. That allows enough time for the important physiological adaptations to take place; or conversely, for factors calling for discontinuance of exercise to make their appearance. If you decide to try the 1½-mile run, pay close attention to the following rules:

1. Do not run to complete exhaustion; use some caution in deciding how hard to push yourself. Do not take the test competitively under any circumstances; let others do what they will while you set your own pace.

2. Don't try too fast a pace at the start, which will lead to early fatigue. Prepare for the run with some practice or instruction in setting an even pace over the one-and-a-half-mile distance.

3. On the day of the test, refrain from physical exertion, do not smoke, and eat nothing for two hours before the run.

4. Precede the test with ten or fifteen minutes of warm-up exercises (Chapter 9).

5. Time the run in minutes and seconds by a clock or stopwatch. *Don't end with a sprint!*

6. At the end of the run, continue walking for another five minutes or so to cool off. The walking enhances venous blood return to the heart and avoids pooling of the blood in the lower extremities, thus aiding in cardiovascular recovery.

The following table shows how time relates to physical fitness in men of various ages. At the present writing there are not enough available data for women.

RATINGS FOR 1½-MILE RUN
(Time in minutes & seconds)
(Men)

Age:	Under 30	Under 40	Under 50	50 & Over
Excellent	10:00–10:30	10:30–11:00	11:30–12:00	12:30–13:00
Good	11:00–11:30	11:30–12:00	12:00–13:00	13:30–14:00
Average	12:00–14:00	13:00–15:00	14:00–16:00	15:00–17:00
Fair	14:30–15:00	16:00–16:30	17:00–17:30	18:00–18:30
Poor	15:30–16:00	17:00–17:30	18:00–18:30	19:00–19:30

Summing Up

The purpose of all these tests, of course, is to create a comprehensive statistical picture of physical fitness, which can be used to measure progress and to modify your continuing exercise program. The tests are non-competitive and definitely should not be approached as a competition race. The norms of performance for various ages given in this chapter simply put an individual performance in perspective. You know by these ratings whether your scores are average, better than average, or not as good as average. You then have a clear guide to the areas where exercise will do you the most good.

While some sophisticated tests require equipment not ordinarily available outside of a YMCA or a laboratory, those described in this chapter suffice for a basic fitness evaluation. The results should be recorded and dated. The tests may be repeated from time to time as a measure of progress. Use a simple record form like this:

PHYSICAL FITNESS EVALUATION

Name _____ Date _____ Age _____
Weight_____lbs. Resting Heart Rate_____/min.
Ideal Weight_____lbs.
Difference _____lbs.
(*Note:* Your actual weight should be within 10 percent of your ideal weight.)
Blood Pressure: Systolic_____/ Diastolic_____
(*Note:* Values over 140/90 are considered high, and any below 110/65 are considered low blood pressure. Values exceeding 160/95 are labeled as hypertensive.)

TEST RESULTS

Test	Page	Your Score	Average for Age	Rating (Good, Fair, etc.)
Body Composition (percent body fat)	59	_____%	_____%	_____
3-Minute Step Test (heart rate)	101	_____bpm	_____bpm	_____
Trunk Flexion (reach in inches)	102	_____in.	_____in.	_____

Hand Grip Strength (kilograms)	104	_____k.g.	_____kg.	_____
1-Minute Sit-Ups (number)	105	_____	_____	_____
12-Minute Distance (miles)	108	_____mi.	_____mi.	_____
1½-Mile Run (minutes, seconds)	109	_____min.:sec	_____min.:sec.	_____

Maybe You Don't Need Tests

Let it be stated flatly that *most people* can undertake a moderate, regulated physical fitness program such as walking or swimming without risk and without taking a fitness test of any kind. As a matter of fact, fitness tests are *not recommended* for totally non-conditioned persons, especially those over 40, because of the danger of their pushing themselves too hard.

Caution is certainly advisable before tackling the more strenuous activities such as jogging or running for the sake of quicker training effects.

Chapter 9

HOW TO EXERCISE

An exercise program properly planned consists of three stages—and it is vital to include all three in your exercise regime. The three stages are (1) the warm-up, getting ready for vigorous exertion; (2) the peak exertion, aimed at achieving a training effect; and (3) the cooling-off, to return the body to normal. This three-way division applies not only to a complete fitness program covering two or three months but to each single session of exercise, such as an hour in the gym.

Impatient people often overlook or slight numbers 1 and 3, the warming-up and cooling-off stages. They want to get right to the nub of exercising, get their muscles vibrating, and get back to their regular routine without delay. Similarly, they may feel they are ready for a fast game of tennis after no more preparation than getting out of the car and walking over to the court. And at the conclusion of a game or exercise session they may feel that all they need is a shower to be ready for normal workaday activity.

Such an approach not only defeats the purpose of body conditioning but may be actually harmful or even hazardous to health, especially for unfit adults over 35. Prudent planning of your exercise program should include leisurely warm-ups as the body adjusts to exercise and adequate time to cool off and return to normal resting state.

The connective tissue of middle-aged persons is usually less elastic than in former years; it needs careful pre-adaptation through stretching. In a person of any age who has been inactive, sudden exertion can produce strains and pain unless attention has been paid to heating up the body to accelerate metabolism, stretch tight ligaments and connective collagen tissue, lubricate creaky joints, stimulate heart and lung action, and sharpen muscular coordination.

During the first three weeks of a fitness program, *all* exercises should be of this warm-up quality, gradually increasing in intensity until the body is ready for heavier activity and peak energy output.

Exercise Opportunities in Daily Life

It appears to be human nature to do things the easy way whenever there is a choice. With physical fitness your goal, you should resist this tendency by making up your mind *not* to take the easy way every time. Grasp each opportunity to exercise your muscles, heart, and lungs even if you are nowhere near a gymnasium or athletic field. Develop a vigorous pattern of living, starting with the way you get out of bed in the morning.

Sleep on a firm mattress, especially if you have experienced twinges of back pain. When you awake, stretch vigorously, squeeze the knees to the chest. Extend the legs to the ceiling, move your legs in cycling fashion. Then climb out of bed and do a few arm swinging and body rotation exercises. These motions are aids to circulation and relieve muscle tension.

Always stand up while dressing (or undressing). Tie shoelaces with feet on the floor rather than putting one foot on a chair. Bend the knees as you reach down.

If you drive a car to work, deliberately park it a half mile to a mile from your destination, and walk the rest of the way. Using public transportation, walk to the next bus stop or transit station rather than patronize the nearest one to home, and get off one stop too soon.

If you must carry a briefcase or shoulder bag, alternately shift the load from side to side.

Leave an elevator two floors too soon and climb the stairs the rest of the way. When returning, walk down three floors or more; it stretches the leg muscles.

Don't jump in the car for every little errand: ride shank's mare whenever you can. Walk down to the post office, walk to the store to pick up the Sunday paper, etc. It's easier to persuade yourself to walk when you have a goal. Remember, at the same time you are wasting gasoline you are also wasting health and fitness. Leave the car at home—perhaps the best single piece of health advice in this book.

114

After a bath or shower, do a brief workout with the towel. Hold it around the small of the back; push against the towel by tightening the muscles of the abdomen and buttocks. Repeat with the towel around the nape of the neck; push against it with neck and chin. Finally, hold the towel like a sling; alternately push each foot by the tips of the toes into the towel while pulling up on it.

Exercise while doing housework. It will be more fun and less fatiguing. When standing at a counter to prepare food or at the sink to wash dishes, rise up and down on the toes. It strengthens ankle and calf muscles. Tighten the abdominal muscles constantly until it becomes a reflex or automatic motion.

Pick up things from the floor with a crisscross motion: use your right arm to pick up an item that's close to your left foot, and vice versa. This stretches muscles of the lower back and thighs.

If you work at a desk, stand up after each phone call and pull in your abdomen sharply—but do not hold your breath. Walk around the room or to the water cooler and stretch before sitting down again.

While seated, occasionally raise both legs from the floor and hold them up for a few seconds. Alternately point the toes and curl toes toward you, while stretching the legs as far as possible. Then lower the legs slowly to the floor.

Seat yourself in a chair by backing into it, then bending the knees. Don't fall into a chair or sprawl. To get up, place feet under the seat and push against the floor.

Take a deep breath once in a while, and exhale forcibly. Unless you are in a room full of smokers, the air indoors is just as good for this purpose as outdoor air.

Rotate your shoulders backward in a shrugging motion to stretch the muscles of the chest and discourage "round shoulders."

Sit tall and straight, hips against the back of the chair, feet flat on the floor. Lean forward from the hips, keeping the back straight. Don't cross the legs, which retards circulation. Keep the chin back to improve both sitting and standing posture.

To lift anything, don't bend the back, bend the knees. With one foot forward for balance, get as close to the object as possible, go into a deep knee-bend, and lift in a vertical line by straightening the legs. Raise a window by standing close to it and lift with elbows bent, feet pushing against the floor. This technique avoids spine strain and so-called sacro-iliac trouble.

Walk with regard to good posture: back straight, head high, legs swinging freely from hips. Swing the arms and keep feet pointing straight ahead.

Climb stairs with body erect, and if possible, maintain balance without using the handrail. Place weight on the ball of the foot rather than on the toes. When you stop to rest, keep moving about the landing or stretch, rather than relaxing completely. Running upstairs two at a time is vigorous exercise.

When obliged to stand at work or when waiting for some-one, stand tall and evenly balanced with weight on heels and outer sides of the feet. Rock from heels to toes or press the toes against the floor, and straighten posture by pressing back against a wall or post.

Social dancing is fine exercise, mild to moderate in ball-room dancing, moderate to strenuous in square dancing and folk dancing. The girl in the song who "could have danced all night" would have had herself a pretty good workout along with the romance.

What about Sports?

Games and sports, whether competitive or solo, may be great fun—but not many are recommended by physical fitness experts as a means of developing endurance and strength. The few exceptions include strenuous swimming and hand-ball.

The problem with most sports is that activity is sporadic. Such sports do not provide the continuous, rhythmic activity that strengthens heart and lung action or promotes muscle flexibility. The exertion is merely incidental to practicing a skill.

Thus some popular sports, including bowling, golf, and archery, contribute little to physical fitness but are desirable for relaxation, enjoyment, and relief of stress. Others, such as handball and soccer, are almost *too* strenuous unless one plays the game two or three times weekly. The unfit Sunday athlete, like the Sunday driver, may be taking his life in his hands.

Most persons seeking to participate in sports should do some physical training *for* the game rather than expect the game to provide the training. Professional athletes don't just run out on a field to play football or baseball. They undergo an intensive conditioning program that begins some weeks before the season opens. They also warm up with calisthenics, running, or practice of their particular skills just before each game begins.

One of the great benefits of a body conditioning program comes with becoming more adept at one's favorite sports. The warm-up exercises and beginner's exercise program in this and the next chapters could be your secret weapon the next time you join a foursome for golf or swing a bat at a fast ball, high outside.

Setting Up an Exercise Program

The recommended schedule for a fitness program would include *a minimum of forty to forty-five minutes of exercising three times a week*. The complete YMCA program for beginners—that is, for anyone not already in fit physical condition—covers ten weeks.

In the early weeks, fifteen minutes, or even more, are devoted to warm-up exercises and ten minutes to cooling-off exercises (warm-up in reverse). This leaves fifteen to twenty minutes for strength, flexibility, and cardiovascular endurance exercises, or "peak work." The proportions change as the program progresses. The time allotted to warm-up and cooldown decreases or, rather, is transferred to the central or "business" part of the exercises. (See chart, page 150.)

Of course, these time allotments may be followed in principle without necessarily adhering to stopwatch exactitude. During the early weeks a greater amount of time is devoted to warm-up because it can be taken for granted that the person starting an exercise program will be in generally poor condition. For such persons, the simple warm-up exercises given in this chapter will add up to enough stress to help produce a cardiovascular training effect, even if nothing more intensive is done for a while.

Warm-up Principles

Certain principles are followed in selecting warm-up exercises. They should be taken *in the sequence* given here and for the length of time or number of repetitions specified. The sequence is designed to accomplish these desired health results:

1. A gradual increase in the intensity of exercise as the warm-up progresses.
2. Exercises that stretch muscles and put joints through their full range of motion, but do not strain them against resistance.
3. Exercises that are rhythmic in nature with a natural flow from one to the next (and avoidance of sudden changes and breaks).
4. Variety to make the warm-up more enjoyable, on the simple concept that body motion is fun—let's make it so.
5. A combination of muscle stretching with increased activity of the heart and vascular system.
6. Inclusion of all segments of the body and all natural motions: the neck, shoulder girdle, shoulder joints, trunk, hip joints, knees (especially to stretch the hamstring muscles behind the knees), and ankles (especially to stretch the calves).

These motions are technically described as *flexion* (bending), *extension* (stretching), *rotation* (as of the neck), *elevation* (as of the shoulder girdle), *abduction* and *adduction* (drawing away and pulling together, as in raising and lowering the arms), and *circumduction* (circular motion, as of the hips, trunk, or shoulders).

Note: While the exact order of engaging the various muscles does not appear to be crucial, some authorities empirically recommend in sequence: (1) shoulders, (2) hip and spine, (3) knees, (4) neck, (5) ankle and foot.

It is also important when beginning the exercises not to eat for an hour or two beforehand, not to smoke (definitely!), and to refrain from alcohol for at least four hours. Drinking causes a constriction of the coronary arteries of the heart just when exercise will increase the oxygen demands of the heart, calling for dilatation (increased opening) rather than constriction of these blood vessels.

As a preparation for cardiovascular training activity such

as running or jogging, the function of the warm-up is to help meet the increased demand for oxygen by the heart, lungs, and active muscles. Specifically, the small blood vessels are opened up not only in the heart's coronary circulation but in the peripheral capillary circulation of the legs and other areas of the body. The warm-up also stretches certain leg muscles exerted in jogging.

A typical warm-up sequence should include two divisions: walking warm-up for eight to ten minutes, and standing warm-up for six to eight minutes.

Walking Warm-up   Total time: 8–9 minutes

1. Main Street Stroll   30 seconds

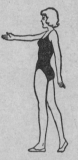

Walk with long strides for a fast pace, swinging arms briskly in rhythm with walk. For promoting general circulation.

2. Forward Crawl Stroke   20 seconds

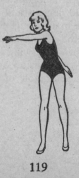

Bend slightly forward at waist and rotate arms alternately in large circles from shoulder joints, similar to the crawl stroke in swimming. For abduction and adduction of shoulder girdle; forward rotation, extension, circumduction, and general loosening of shoulder joints. May be done while walking or in standing position.

3. Arm Pumping   *15 seconds*

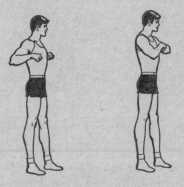

Walk with pumping arms, in four counts at a moderate rate. Counts 1, 2, 3 consist of holding elbows bent to approximately 90 degrees and then swinging them back vigorously while maintaining the elbow angle (3 counts per step). On the fourth count, allow the elbows to extend and the arms to swing backward freely (1 count per 2 steps). For extension and hyperextension at the shoulder joints, adduction of shoulder girdle.

4. *Side-to-Side Stretch*   *15 seconds*

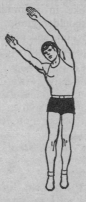

Raise hands together overhead and bend from side to side in rhythm with walking steps. Bend to the side of the leg swinging forward; for example, when stepping out with left leg, stretch to the left. For stretching of lateral trunk muscles. May also be done while standing.

5. *Walk with a Twist*   *15 seconds*

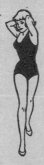

Clasp hands behind the head and twist from side to side in rhythm with walking steps. Twist the body to the same side as the leg swinging forward. For general circulation, rotation of trunk, abduction, adduction, and elevation of shoulder girdle.

6. *Repeat Main Street Stroll*   **15 *seconds***
Gradually increase pace up to a jog.

7. *Jog*   **30 *seconds***
Take a slow pace of ten or twelve minutes per mile around the outside rim of the gymnasium. When jogging (or running), raise knees forward and upward and keep arms close to body, elbows bent. Hold chest up and lean slightly forward, "pumping" with both arms and legs for forcible drive and balance. Run on entire foot, not on the toes. For general increase in circulation and preparation for specific cardiovascular training to come.

8. *Repeat Main Street Stroll*   **15 *seconds***
Ease pace down from jog to walk, a cooling-down or tapering-off maneuver.

9. *Repeat Arm Pumping, Side-to-Side Stretch, Walk with a Twist, Main Street Stroll (Nos. 3 to 6)*   **60 *seconds***

10. *Jog*   **60 *seconds***

11. *Repeat Main Street Stroll*   **15 *seconds***

12. *Repeat Nos. 3 to 6*   **60 *seconds***

13. *Jog*   **90 *seconds***

14. *Repeat Main Street Stroll*   **15 *seconds***

15. *Repeat Nos. 3 to 6*   **60 *seconds***
End in position for standing warm-up.

Standing Warm-up   Total time: 7–8 minutes

1. *Arm Circles*   **20–30 *seconds***

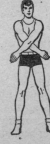

Move the arms so that the shoulder joint turns through a 360-degree rotation in a vertical plane, and again in a horizontal plane. To do this, swing both hands together up and down, then from side to side across chest. Breathe freely and exhale forcibly as each arm reaches the bottom end of the rotation.

2. *Repeat Crawl Stroke Forward*
   (standing)   20–30 *seconds*
3. *Repeat Side-to-Side Stretch*
   (standing)   20–30 *seconds*
4. *Crawl Stroke Backward*   20–30 *seconds*

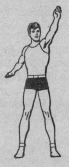

Stand erect. Same as Crawl Stroke Forward, but in reverse direction of rotation, bending slightly rearward from waist. Has effects similar to Crawl Stroke Forward but on different muscles.

The above are a continuation of the general stretching in the Walking Warm-up, but following them come specific stretching exercises. In these, take it easy! Stretch in an easy manner at the beginning. Place emphasis on movement *through the full range of motion*—not on trying to complete the exercise at a fast pace or in more repetitions. A slow pace with full motion will do much more for you.

Whenever the trunk is bent, the knees should be bent also to prevent undue back strain. Never make jerky or sudden movements and don't try to force a muscle beyond the point it seems to want to go. It will stretch further as your training continues; time is on your side! Follow a natural breathing rhythm, too.

5. *Touch Floor and Stretch*   *30 seconds*

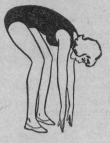

Bend forward with knees slightly bent and touch the floor with fingertips. Bounce slightly from the contact, and repeat for a total of three contacts; on the fourth count, straighten up, extend the back, and stretch (i.e., bounce [easy], bounce, bounce, stretch). Repeat five to ten times. This exercise stretches the hip and back extensor muscles.

6. *Butterfly Stroke*   *20–30 seconds*

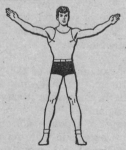

With feet a few inches apart, bend forward slightly and rotate both arms forward simultaneously—something like the butterfly stroke in swimming. For adduction and abduction of shoulder girdle, forward rotation of shoulder joints.

7. *Neck Rotation*   *5 to left, 5 to right*

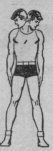

Rotate head fully to the left around the vertical axis. Reverse direction to the right after five repetitions. Exhale when in forward position. For limbering up the vertebrae and muscles of the neck and spine.

8. *Alternate Knee Hug*   *10 times*

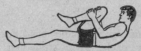

Lie on the back. Lift left knee to the chest, press close to chest with hands with moderate force. Exhale and straighten leg. Repeat with right knee. Try not to raise the buttocks or unused leg from floor while hugging the knee. For stretching the back muscles.

9. *Body Rotation*   *5 to left, 5 to right*

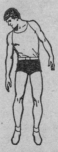

Stand erect but very relaxed. Allow head and shoulders to fall back loosely, bending a little from the waist.

125

Then rotate trunk to the right, allowing the upper body's motion to be accelerated by gravity. Bend the waist forward in a relaxed manner and continue movement around and upward until first position is regained. For stretching muscles of the trunk.

10. *Bending Forward and Back*   *10 times*

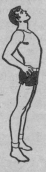

Place hands on hips and bend forward at waist to stretch the back. Then straighten and stretch with shoulders thrown back. For flexion and extension of trunk, some extension of hamstring muscles of the thigh.

11. *Alternate Toe Touch*   *10 times*

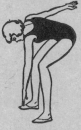

Bend the knees as much as necessary and touch the left foot with the right hand. Without straightening up, twist and touch the right toe with the left hand. Don't try to do this during warm-up without bending the knees. For trunk rotation, stretching of trunk extensors and thigh extensors.

Warm-up for Jogging

The Standing Warm-up may be continued if desired in order to concentrate on particular muscles. The following exercises are especially good if you intend to do any jogging or running. For variety's sake, they may be substituted occasionally for any of the exercises in the suggested program above.

12. *Single Leg Raises*   5 *left, 5 right*

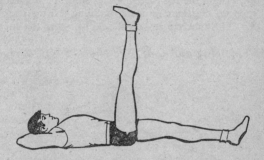

Lie on back with hands folded under head. Lift left leg, hold it straight up, then return leg to within four inches of the floor. Repeat five times, then shift to right leg for five repetitions. This stretches the muscles that flex the knee and extend the hip.

13. *Thigh and Leg Stretcher*   2 *left, 2 right*

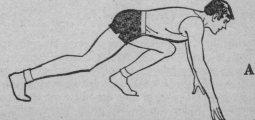

A

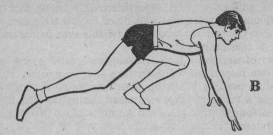

B

Assume sprinter's position on toes as in (A). Lower hips to the floor without shifting position of feet. The stretch should be felt in the anterior (frontal) thigh; if not, extend the leg further back. Repeat for each thigh. Then do the exercise again, pointing the toe back as in (B). This time the stretch should be felt in the shin.

14. Hamstring and Calf Stretcher 2 left, 2 right

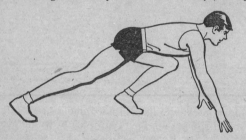

The same as thigh and leg stretcher, but keep the ankle of extended leg dorsi-flexed (point the heel). In this position, the stretch should be felt in the calf muscles, including the hamstrings just behind the knee.

Setting Your Own Pace

During the first weeks of an exercise program the simple warm-up exercises in this chapter provide enough stress for anyone in poor condition to tolerate, and at the same time enough to produce a cardiovascular training effect. Persons who are over 60 years old, or are obese, or have high blood pressure, or suffer from orthopedic problems should not exercise without medical supervision. It may be that pre-conditioning by means of a walking or bicycle ergometer program (see Chapter 11) would be advisable even *before* undertaking a calisthenic warm-up.

Signs of overstress include excessive breathing and poor heart rate response. Frequently take your own pulse, as described on page 91. Note the pulse rate during recovery and use it as a guide. A heart rate taken during the first fifteen seconds following exercise will be quite close to the target heart rate or "exercise value."

An acceptable target heart rate for apparently healthy persons is about 80 percent of the average maximum heart rate estimated for a person's age (i.e., 220 minus age in years). The 80 percent value is equivalent to an energy expenditure of approximately 50 percent of the maximum oxygen intake. The following heart rates approximate this 80 percent–50 percent range as a control of the intensity of exercises you undertake.

TARGET HEART RATES IN EXERCISE

Age	Heart Rate (beats per min.)
20–29	170
30–39	160
40–49	150
50–59	140

Other warning signals include undue fatigue during exercise, inability to recover from a workout throughout the day, inability to sleep at night, and persistent muscle aches and pains. These signs do not, however, preclude *all* exercise. They simply suggest a reduced level of activity until you develop the capacity to handle more intense workouts.

A brisk walking or bicycle ergometer program, as suggested above and described in later chapters, or swimming are suitable for most people because in these activities the intensity can be readily controlled. You do as much as you can, but no more, and quit while you're ahead!

Strength and muscle endurance exercises are planned as an extension of the warm-up—the same types of stretching exercises but progressively more strenuous. The peak-work phase of the YMCA physical fitness program is outlined in the next chapter.

Chapter 10

REACHING A PEAK THE Y'S WAY

A second segment of the three-cycle exercise program develops out of the warm-up segment by escalating the intensity of familiar exercises and employing some new exercises. The objective is to build up to *peak work*—the best a person can do in his present state of body conditioning. He should have a good workout, but not be pushed to exhaustion. In the YMCA suggested program, this segment consists of two types of training: (a) exercises for muscular strength, flexibility, and endurance; and (b) exercises for cardiovascular and respiratory training.

In the first type, calisthenics are selected to provide moderate resistance to muscular contractions, in order to build up strength and agility to a target level. Although an extremely valuable effect in itself, the musculoskeletal training also may be considered a preparation for the cardiovascular work that follows it.

You might be eager to start running now for the sake of your heart and lungs, but remember that you run on legs and feet. Don't neglect them. The musculoskeletal system consists of tissues which require specific stretching and stimulation if they are to perform well on a jog.

Since the muscular buildup exercises constitute a fairly intensive effort, the YMCA has established a few guidelines, which, if observed, will produce best results.

Calisthenic Guidelines

1. Avoid working without letup. Work, then rest, then resume work, and so on. The adult body can adapt to effort

if a rest period permits it to accommodate to exercise before starting again.

2. Avoid isometric (static) exercises, which cause resistance to blood flow. Keep in motion, but don't turn an exercise such as push-ups, into a trial against exhaustion. If the goal is ten push-ups, break them into two separated sets of five instead of one continuous set of ten.

3. Avoid freely swinging the body against a fixed joint. For example, if you can't touch your toes while the knees are locked with legs straight, don't try to force the issue by forceful bouncing downward. The consequence might be a strained back muscle, tendon, or ligament. Instead, bend the knees. Just keep exerting steady force against resistance and eventually you will reach your goal without strain. (Or perhaps the problem is first to eliminate that spare tire around the middle.)

4. In your calisthenic program try to include exercises for all major joint movements, just as in the warm-up series. Plan a specific set of calisthenics, including the number of repetitions, and stick to it. (The YMCA suggested program in this chapter may be used as a guide.)

5. Keep shifting forceful work from one muscle group to another to avoid local fatigue. Don't do more than two consecutive abdominal or two consecutive leg exercises; try something else in between.

6. Don't overwork to exhaustion, but do push yourself far enough for a healthy training effect. Usually this is best accomplished by going through the full range of motion in each exercise. If arms are to be raised overhead, raise them as high as you can; if shoulders are thrown back, throw them all the way back, and so forth. Don't compromise; don't make half-hearted motions. Expect some temporary muscular ache as a sign that you are placing new demands on previously inactive muscle fibers.

7. When working in a group, don't try to keep up with the fittest members if beyond your present capability.

YMCA Muscular Strength and Flexibility Exercises

Total time: about 8 minutes

1. Alternate Knee-Bend Kicks

20 times

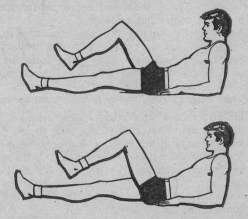

Half-sit, half-lie on the floor, resting weight on the buttocks and forearms. Lean back and raise the heels about four inches off the floor. Flex and extend each leg in turn. You can regulate the difficulty of the exercise by the distance the legs are lifted from the floor. This is training for the abdominal muscles.

2. Short Leg Raises (right)

10 times

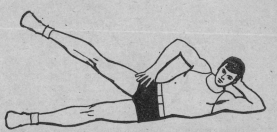

Lying on the left side, support the head on left elbow and place other hand on hip. Head should be in line with spine. Raise the right leg laterally (upward) about

six to eight inches while keeping the knee straight
Lower the leg and repeat. Stretches side muscles of th
thighs.

3. *Flutter Kick on Back*   20 *seconds*

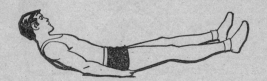

Lie on the back with hands placed, palm down, under
the buttocks. The small of the back should touch the
floor throughout the exercise. Raise the head from the
floor, also extend and raise the legs. Alternately flex
and extend each leg from the hip, but do not touch
the floor. The difficulty may be regulated by the distance the legs are raised from the floor. For the abdominal muscles.

4. *Short Leg Raises (left)*   10 *times*

Same as No. 2, but for the left leg.

5. *Modified Push-ups*   6 *times*

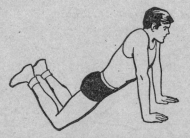

Assume position shown, supporting body weight on
hands and knees. Hands should be placed directly below the shoulders, with body held straight. Lower the
body by bending arms until chest is approximately one

inch from floor. Return to original position by straightening arms. For muscles on back of arms and front of chest.

Note: After the first few weeks, substitute the more difficult Regular Push-ups (page 141).

6. *Shoulder Squeezers*   5 *times*

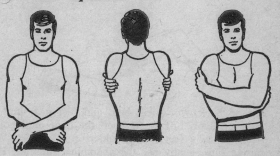

Swing the arms across the front of the body and around the sides as far back as possible. Grasp the shoulders with the hands as if trying to force the shoulder joints together in front. Swing the arms forward again and repeat. For the upper back muscles and shoulder girdle.

7. *Modified Sit-ups*   6 *times*

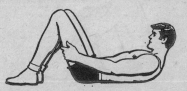

Lie on back with knees flexed to about 90 degrees and feet flat on floor. Rise forward toward a sitting position and grasp the thighs on the sides. Use this leverage to help sit upright. First bend the body at the neck, then at the trunk; roll up into position. A good workout for abdominal muscles.

Note: After the first few weeks, as your body becomes more supple, you may switch to the somewhat more difficult Regular Sit-ups (page 140).

8. Hip Raising 3 times

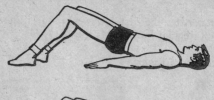

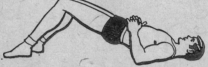

Lie on back with knees bent and feet near buttocks, arms on floor. Lift the hips off the floor until body is straight, using feet and shoulders for support. While raising hips, gently pat the abdominal muscles. Helps recovery of the abdominal muscles after sit-ups; also exercises the back, buttocks, and back of thighs.

9. Sitting Tucks 6 times

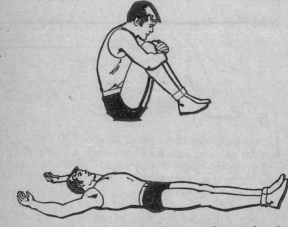

Sitting on the floor, bring knees to chest and tuck them in close with arms and hands clasping shins. Lift feet from floor. Release knees and stretch out supine with arms on the floor overhead. Sit up to repeat the tuck. Exercises abdominal muscles.

10. *Hurdler's Stretch*   *10 times*

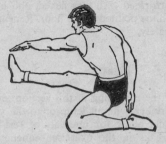

On the floor, assume the position illustrated, which resembles a runner going over a hurdle. Start with right leg extended and left leg folded under buttock. Reach forward and touch the right foot with the left hand. Repeat five times, moving slowly and in a relaxed manner (do not bounce). Then gently stretch backward. Switch leg and arm positions to the other side for five more repetitions. Stretches the lower limbs in preparation for jogging.

11. *Thigh Stretcher*   *6 times*

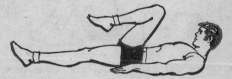

Lie on floor with legs extended. Flex knee and thigh of one leg and bring up to chest. Then, keeping the ankle plantar flexed (pointing the toe), extend the knee and thigh toward the ceiling, then slowly lower leg to floor. Repeat three times with each leg. Another warm-up exercise for jogging.

Two other exercises may be borrowed from the warm-up series as further preparation for jogging. The Hamstring and Calf Stretcher (page 128) may be done six times, or three for each leg; the stretch should be felt in the calf muscles. The Thigh and Leg Stretcher (page 127) is felt in front of the thigh when performed with toes flexed, and in the shin when performed with toe pointed to the floor. Repeat three times for each leg alternately.

Time Out for Rest

As stated at the beginning of this section, exercising should never be undertaken without letup or to the point of exhaustion. One should allow for intervals of rest wherever there are natural breaks in the exercise sequence, for example, following calisthenics such as the muscle-training series, and before starting to jog or run for cardiovascular training.

Physiologically, there is a proper way to rest, which is illustrated and described below. The heart rate should drop below 110–120 beats per minute before resuming work. Assuming the correct rest position helps in recovery of the heart and lungs and in easing any muscle tensions after a brisk workout.

12. Recovery Rest   *2–3 minutes*

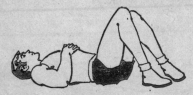

Lie supine, flat on the back, with knees bent and feet apart with heels *out* and toes turned *in*. The position may be modified by head and neck rotation to help muscles relax.

Other Muscle-Training Exercises

The preceding series completes a well-rounded program of muscle training and should be followed by the suggested few minutes of supine rest. For variety, or to engage still other muscles, any of the following group may be added to or substituted in the sequence.

13. *Flutter Kicks on Front*   20 *seconds*

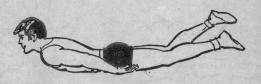

Lie prone with hands at sides (or you may rest the chin on hands held palms down). With knees extended, alternately kick legs as in swimming, with feet moving about six inches. For muscles of the back, buttocks, and posterior thighs.

14. *Half Squats*   10 *times*

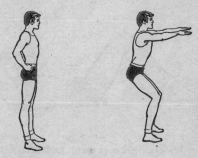

Stand with hands on hips. Lower body to half-squat (or partial knee-bend) position while thrusting arms forward. Return to original position and repeat with rhythmic motions. For calves, thighs, and buttocks.

15. Bent-Knee Leg Raises   10 times

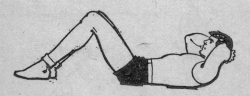

Lie on back and hold right knee with hands. Lift left leg to vertical position and return to within four inches of the floor. Repeat five times with left leg then switch to right leg for five repetitions. An abdominal exercise.

16. Regular Sit-up   6 times

Lie on back with knees bent and feet flat on floor as for Modified Sit-up (page 135), but clasp hands behind neck and complete sitting upright without using hands for leverage. Then continue by twisting the trunk to touch each elbow in turn to the opposite knee. Remember to *roll* up by bending the neck first, then the trunk. For abdominal muscles.

140

17. *Regular Push-up*　　　　　　　*6 times*

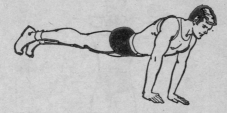

Assume position shown, with body supported by hands
and toes, legs and body held straight, and hands placed
below the shoulders. Lower body to within one inch
of the floor and return without bending hips or knees.
A back and abdominal exercise, but also specifically
develops triceps muscle of the upper arm.

18. *Hands and Heels Stretch*　　　　*6 times*

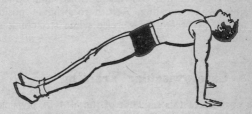

Lie on back with hands on floor pointed backward.
Raise body and arch back upward. Return to position
with head and body straight, and repeat. For stretching
the back muscles.

19. Breast Stroke   6 times

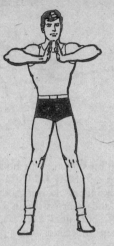

Stand with feet shoulder-width apart and hands together in front of chest, elbows held at shoulder height.
Then raise arms outward and upward while inhaling.
Now allow arms to swing outward and downward to
sides while exhaling. Return to original position and
repeat. A breathing exercise while stretching shoulder
muscles.

YMCA Cardiovascular Training

The purpose of this segment of the YMCA physical fitness
program for beginners is to produce beneficial training effects in the heart, arteries, lungs, and other elements of the
circulatory and respiratory systems of the body. Essentially
it consists of walking, jogging, and running under controlled
conditions, combined with stretching and flexibility exercises
to facilitate warming up and cooling down.

Running tends to stiffen the muscles and ligaments of the
spine and legs if you are not in condition. Therefore, it is
wise to prepare the muscles for jogging and to taper off with
tension-relaxing calisthenics.

Among the simplest and most effective of tension-easing exercises is just plain walking. Never abruptly stop a jog or a run, but continue for three minutes or so walking and stretching. Gradually bring the body functions back to near resting conditions, with heart rate below 110–120.

How to Jog

You should take a minute or two to master the mechanics of jogging and running. Run with either a heel-and-toe or flat-footed strike where the foot meets the track. Avoid a footstrike on the ball of the foot or on the toes. Run with a forward rolling motion and push-off. A proper technique will protect the feet and the rest of the skeleton from shocks, strains, and jarring.

If you jog around the track of a typical gym, alternate the direction from counterclockwise to clockwise and vice versa. This prevents stress on one side of the body caused by continually leaning one way into the turns.

Clothes are important, too. Don't try to "work up a sweat" with rubberized or other impervious garments. You'll work up a sweat soon enough in ordinary running pants and a T-shirt. "Sweat" clothes may easily get you overheated. Be especially careful in hot weather (see page 77).

Good shoes are a must if one is to avoid leg soreness, and good socks keep the feet dry and avoid blisters. There are, of course, many brands of athletic footwear and the advice of a physical director at your gym probably should be followed.

Generally, you get what you pay for. A first-class outfit, though it may cost more than the cheapest, will be a good investment in your health. Discard shoes that are obviously worn out or lopsided. Running shoes should have a thick sole and be cushioned in the heel, to protect the Achilles tendon from strain, and prevent bruising of the heel.

Jogging Guidelines

In a beginner's program, the recommended exercise intensity for the cardiovascular segment is to jog at a pace of one mile in ten minutes. This may be too fast for you at first, especially if you are in very poor condition. When jogging take a 10-second reading of your pulse from time to time; the heart rate should stay within the age-adjusted limits suggested previously.

Breathe normally as you run, but accentuate the exhaling. Ordinarily, exhale on effort. *Do not hold the breath.*

The 10-minute-per-mile pace will be maintained throughout the entire ten-week program. You may wonder, then, how you can improve or at least continue to get a training effect if you do not increase the work load with a faster pace. The load does increase because in the YMCA program jogging occurs in *sets*.

Each set consists in part of jogging, in part of recovery by slowing down to a walk, and the proportions are variable. Thus, you might start with a 1-minute set (one minute of jogging, two minutes of recovery) and a few weeks later progress to a 3-minute set (three minutes of jogging, two minutes of recovery). The weekly progression schedule on page 150 shows how work loads are judiciously increased.

In exercising your heart and lungs, realize that you are exercising *muscles*. The heart is one of the strongest muscles in the body and is worked the hardest. Just as in conditioning other muscles of the body, the *interval principle* of alternating work and rest should be obeyed. Each person must limit the intensity of exercise to his own capabilities, using the technique of heart rate monitoring (frequently taking the pulse) to keep himself within physiological limits.

Jogging and running are companionable sports; it's always more fun to run in a group. But don't let companionship metamorphose into competition. If you are very unfit or obese, hard running can be dangerous. Stick to your own pace. Let time and regularity of workouts build you up until you can run for longer distances and enjoy group running.

YMCA Exercise Program for Heart and Lungs

Total time: 8½ min.

1. Main Street Stroll (page 119)   30 seconds

This warm-up exercise is peculiarly suited to cardiac-respiratory work. It consumes more energy than ordinary walking in the street and is more specifically aimed at stretching the muscles.

2. Jog   1 minute

Maintain 10-minutes-per-mile pace. You can ascertain the proper pace by finding the length of a lap and timing one circuit with a stopwatch; correct the pace if too fast or too slow. (See lap conversion chart on page 146.) Check your footstrike; make sure to run in heel-toe or flat-footed style, not on the toes. Reverse direction of run at least once to balance stresses in circular running.

3. Arm Pumping (page 120)   20 seconds

This exercise and the next three maneuvers are helpful in recovery from jogging. Do them vigorously and *keep walking*. Take your pulse during this recovery interval and decide whether to continue jogging or to switch to a walking program.

Converting Time to Laps

Having determined the number of laps per mile in a given gymnasium, jogging time specified in seconds can be converted into number of laps. They may be easier to count than measuring the time. If the pace is to be one mile in ten minutes, the following table provides a basis for conversion.

Laps per mile	Time to run one lap at 10 min./mile pace
18	33 sec.
20	30 sec.
24	25 sec.
27	22 sec.
33	18 sec.

Divide the time allotted for jogging by the number of seconds per lap in the table above. This will give the number of laps to be run in that time at a 10-minute-per-mile pace. Suppose the track measures twenty laps to the mile and you

LAPS PER MILE PER SIZE OF GYM OR FIELD (Length x Width) (For example, in a 30' x 30' gym there will be 64 laps to the mile; in a 50' x 50' gym 33 laps, etc.)

FEET	30	35	40	45	50	55	60	65	70	75	80	85	90	95	100	105	110
30	64	57	52	47	43	40	37	35	33	31	29	27	26	25	24	23	22
35	57	52	47	43	40	37	35	33	31	29	27	26	25	24	23	22	21
40	52	47	43	40	37	35	33	31	29	27	26	25	24	23	22	21	20
45	47	43	40	37	35	33	31	29	27	26	25	24	23	22	21	20	19
50	43	40	37	35	33	31	29	27	26	25	24	23	22	21	20	19	19
55	40	37	35	33	31	29	27	26	25	24	23	22	21	20	19	19	18
60	37	35	33	31	29	27	26	25	24	23	22	21	20	19	19	18	17
65	35	33	31	29	27	26	25	24	23	22	21	20	19	19	18	17	17
70	33	31	29	27	26	25	24	23	22	21	20	19	19	18	17	17	16
75	31	29	27	26	25	24	23	22	21	20	19	19	18	17	17	16	16
80	29	27	26	25	24	23	22	21	20	19	19	18	17	17	16	16	15
85	27	26	25	24	23	22	21	20	19	19	18	17	17	16	16	15	15
90	26	25	24	23	22	21	20	19	19	18	17	17	16	16	15	15	15
95	25	24	23	22	21	20	19	19	18	17	17	16	16	15	15	15	14
100	24	23	22	21	20	19	19	18	17	17	16	16	15	15	15	14	14
105	23	22	21	20	19	19	18	17	17	16	16	15	15	15	14	14	13
110	22	21	20	19	19	18	17	17	16	16	15	15	15	14	14	13	13

are to run one minute (60 seconds). The table shows that on a twenty-lap circuit the time per lap is thirty seconds. Therefore:

$$\frac{60 \text{ seconds}}{30 \text{ sec./lap}} = 2 \text{ laps}$$

In other words, if you run two laps in the one minute allotted, you are maintaining a pace of one mile in ten minutes (on that particular track).

4. *Hands Together Overhead*   *20 seconds*

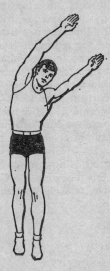

Continue to walk but with arms stretched overhead, swaying slightly from side to side.

5. *Side-to-Side Stretch (page 121)*   *20 seconds*
A natural progression from the previous movement. Assume same position, but emphasize bending and stretching to each side.

6. *Walk with a Twist (page 121)*   *20 seconds*
Again a natural progression from the previous movement—but with emphasis on body rotation.

7. *Repeat Nos. 1 through 6*   *2 min. 50 sec.*
8. *Again repeat Nos. 1 through 6* *2 min. 30 sec.*
   You can accommodate the amount of activity in this recovery period to your present tolerance of exercise by shortening the time given to each unit. But it's better not to omit any.

Cooling-off Period

The cooling-off period comes at the end of your workout —after the calisthenics and running—but being last does not make it least in importance. Its general purpose, of course, is literally to cool off—stop sweating and breathing hard—to return body functions gradually to the pre-exercise level. Physiologically, the exercises used for cooling off are designed to promote the return of blood to the heart from the extremities, with no pooling or Valsalva effect.

Cooling off takes five to ten minutes, more in the early weeks of physical fitness training, less at the end of conditioning. (See the chart on page 150.) At its conclusion, the heart rate should be below 110–120 beats per minute. Whereas in previous exercises the emphasis has been upon vigorous exertion, the emphasis in cooling off is shifted to relaxation and slowing down.

In short, cooling off is a warm-up in reverse. The cooldown exercises in the following YMCA suggested program are of the non-tensive, relaxing type and are performed in a non-stressful fashion.

YMCA Cool-down Exercises   Total time 7–8 minutes

1. *Main Street Stroll (page 119)*   20 *seconds*
2. *Forward Crawl Stroke (page 119)*   20 *seconds*
3. *Side-to-Side Stretch (page 121)*   20 *seconds*
4. *Walk with a Twist (page 121)*   20 *seconds*
5. *Half Jog*   90 *seconds*
   This is a very slow jog without lifting the feet as much as in the regular jog—resembles a shuffle.

6. *Repeat Nos. 1 through 4*	*80*	*seconds*
7. *Half Jog*	*60*	*seconds*
8. *Repeat Nos. 1 through 4*	*80*	*seconds*
9. *Half Jog*	*30*	*seconds*

9. Note that the time devoted to slow jogging has been reduced thirty seconds on each repetition, from one and a half minutes to one minute to a half minute, while the stretching exercises are repeated in full.

10. *Repeat Nos. 1 through 4*	*80*	*seconds*

11. *Main Street Stroll, gradually coming to a stop.*
12. *Take pulse. If over 100 beats per minute, continue walking two or three more laps.*

Stretching exercises performed on the floor, such as that on page 127, are also suitable for cooling off after a run. But do not include any tension exercises such as the Isometric Shoulder Squeeze. A particularly good one is the Upside-Down Bicycle (page 161).

The 10-Week Beginner's Program

Previously in this chapter we have noted that a good body conditioning program will consist of forty to forty-five minutes per exercise session, three times a week. Regularity and *consistency* every second day will make or break your success at achieving physical fitness.

Similar reasoning applies to *continuance* of the program over a period of time. Physical education experts agree that approximately two and a half months, or *ten weeks*, will be necessary to advance the normal unfit beginner into a body condition that will permit him to exercise without discomfort and be ready for the new challenges of a healthy, active life.

In the YMCA 10-week program outlined in the table on page 150, a model progression or gradual increase in the intensity of work is indicated. Here are some points to observe in following this progression.

The total workout time is a close approximation, but can be varied by a minute or two either way, or in each section, without harm. It adds up to about forty minutes at the start of the program, increasing to forty-five minutes or more at the conclusion.

WEEKLY PROGRESSION FOR BEGINNER'S EXERCISE PROGRAM

Week	Warm-up (min.)	Muscular Strength & Endurance				Cardiovascular			Cool-off (min.)	Total Time (min.)
		Push-ups	Shoulder Squeezer	Flutter (sec.)	Sit-ups	Sit Tucks	Time (min.)	Jogging		
1	15	6(M)	5	20	6	6	6	3-1 min. sets	10	40
2	15	8(M)	6	20	7	6	6	3-1½ min. sets	10	40
3	14	10(M)	7	20	8	10	7	3-2 min. sets	9	41
4	14	6	8	25	9	10	7	3-2½ min. sets	9	41
5	13	7	9	25	10	15	8	3-3 min. sets	8	42
6	12	7	10	30	11	15	8	3-3½ min. sets	7	43
7	12	8	10	30	12	20	8	3-4 min. sets	7	43
8	11	8	10	30	13	20	9	3-4½ min. sets	6	44
9	11	9	10	30	14	25	10	3-5 min. sets	6	44
10	10	10	10	30	15	25	10	10 min. mile	5	45

(M) is modified push-up. A jogging set consists of the time listed for jogging followed by 2 min. recovery.

1. *Warm-up period.* As the program progresses, the time allotted for warm-up decreases from fifteen minutes the first week to ten minutes in the last week. However, the pace increases; that is, the same number of warm-up exercises are performed in a shorter time. Experience shows that the improving condition of the participant permits an accelerated pace. After a few weeks, you will feel able to zip through the warm-up without even breathing hard.

The exercises may remain the same from week to week, using the model warm-up session in Chapter 9 as a guide. For the sake of variety and of spreading the training effect to all parts of the body, you may substitute a new exercise every week or two. Choose from the group of stretching exercises on pages 124–128.

2. *Muscular strength, endurance, and flexibility period.* The strength and endurance exercises shown in the table increase in number of repetitions from week to week. But the *stretching* (flexibility) exercises in the model workout (pages 133–137) may be used without change in number of repetitions from week to week. The stretching exercises include Alternate Knee-Bend Kicks (20 times), Short Leg Raises (10 times), Hip Raising (3 times), Hurdler's Stretch (10 times), and Thigh Stretcher (6 times).

Again, it is desirable to add variety. Occasionally substitute exercises from the group beginning on page 139. In body conditioning as in other activities, variety is the spice of life—it adds interest to each new session.

The frequency-intensity for each exercise is shown in the table either as the number of repetitions or the time in seconds. The total time devoted to muscle-building increases from about six minutes the first week to ten minutes in the last week.

All told, the table represents a typical program that might be given to a group of beginners by the physical director of a YMCA. If you are setting up a program for yourself, study the table carefully with reference to the exercise descriptions in this chapter. Note particularly the muscle groups that each exercise affects and try to design a well-rounded body-conditioning program for yourself.

3. *Cardiovascular training period.* The table lists cardiovascular training in jogging sets. A set consists of the time allotted to actual jogging plus two minutes of recovery. Thus, the three one-minute sets of the first week each consists of one

minute of running and two minutes of walking recovery, total three minutes per set—or nine to ten minutes for the three sets in the entire cardiovascular period.

The walking recovery should include exercise movements as in the model C.V. session appearing on pages 142–149. They greatly speed recovery of the heart-pumping system without any of the gasping, heaving, or other distress that might come with a sudden stop.

Note that in the tenth week the upward progression of jogging time to twenty-one minutes in week nine appears to be abruptly reversed to ten minutes for a single mile. But it isn't. Running a complete 10-minute-mile fully replaces the previous sets in terms of oxygen uptake, and for most participants will be quite enough jogging for one day.

4. *Cool-down period.* In summary, the time allotted to muscular exercises and to cardiovascular training steadily increases over the ten-week span. Meanwhile, time allotted to warm-up shrinks, but with the result of increasing its intensity. The time allotted to cool-off shrinks about 50 percent. As your physical condition improves, the less pampering your heart and muscles will need to take the main exertions in stride. A slower heart rate and a happy improvement in your "wind" will mark the change. For cool-down, follow the schedule on pages 148–149.

The Buddy System

In scuba diving, no one is supposed to descend to the depths alone. He dives with a watchful companion who is supposed to keep track of the submerged diver and give assistance when needed. This is known as the "buddy system." Something like it has been used to good effect by YMCA physical directors leading an exercise group.

One of the principal hazards of any program calling for an output of physical effort is a tendency of people to drop out before the hoped-for conditioning has been accomplished. Four reasons for it are obvious: (1) laziness, (2) displeasure, discomfort, or disappointment, (3) preoccupation with other affairs, and (4) inconvenience.

It's very easy to find excuses for skipping an exercise class: business demands, social affairs, distance, the gasoline shortage, just-don't-feel-like-it-today—you name it. Whatever the reason, dropping out for *even one session* retards body conditioning and depreciates your investment in better health. Some people drop out because they feel so good after a few sessions they think the job's done and there's no need for any more. (They're wrong!)

The buddy system in an exercise class works like this. With one other member of the class you form a two-person team. If your friend doesn't show up at the gym one day, you call him up. If *you* don't show up, *he* calls *you*. Answering that call requires a plausible reason, and thinking up new reasons each time gets a bit embarrassing. Not to say tiresome. Each buddy has an incentive to make the class on a regular schedule —avoiding the label of quitter.

Even if right now you feel pretty determined to keep exercising until once again you can make your body obey orders without strain, the extra incentive of being answerable to a buddy won't hurt. If you're training in a group, try it.

The next chapter continues the YMCA program for "graduates" of the beginner's exercise program. The graduation diploma comes with the ability to complete, without undue difficulty, the one-mile jog listed in the previous chart on page 150 for the tenth week.

Also in the next two chapters are special programs for a variety of situations: walking and jogging for the sedentary, cycling and swimming, and ways to prepare for skiing or other sports.

Chapter 11

A POST-GRADUATE COURSE

Completing the beginner's exercise program of ten weeks may call for a celebration. You have graduated to a higher class of the physically fit. Requirement for the diploma: you must be able to jog one mile in ten minutes, the specified cardiovascular training goal for the tenth week.

In the YMCA system, the graduates are ready to begin a second course of exercise, which also covers ten weeks, called the intermediate program. It is "intermediate" because it prepares for still a third, advanced training course at the intensity demanded of athletes or U.S. Marines (and beyond the scope of this book). After intermediate training you should attain a state of fitness enabling you to run two miles in twenty minutes, or exactly twice as far as the graduating beginner.

Now, if at the end of the beginner's ten weeks, you still have difficulty jogging one mile in ten minutes, you should postpone "graduation" indefinitely. Stay with the exercises and the intensities scheduled for the last two weeks of the beginner series. Don't attempt the intermediate level until you can tolerate these last beginner's exercises well.

Deciding how to proceed will depend not only upon your attained degree of physical fitness, but upon your motivation. What do you hope to get out of exercising for your health? If a trim figure and heightened vitality are your only objectives, *you can keep fit on the beginner's program alone.* You don't have to advance to stiffer exertions and a more intense effort. *But you must keep it up!*

Sporadic exercise does little good. Even a brief layoff can cause deterioration to set in. Unfortunately, your body can store fat, but it cannot store fitness. The only way to get the full benefit of physical activity is to maintain the activity—

indefinitely. Look with pride at what you have gained. That feeling of good health is precious. Don't let it slip away.

Assuming you have improved to the point of zipping through the beginner's sessions without much effort, you may be "rarin'" for new mountains to climb. This chapter outlines an intermediate exercise program, and other things you can do to advance fitness, such as systematic jogging.

The calisthenic exercises at the intermediate level are quite similar to those in the beginner's program, in some cases identical. However, the effort required is greater. Week by week, the number of repetitions per exercise is increased or the time for doing them is reduced. Either way, a progressively greater work load is imposed.

Furthermore, where a "modified" (easier) version of certain calisthenics is suggested for beginners, the "regular" (harder) version may be specified for intermediates. These include push-ups, sit-ups, and lateral leg raises.

10-Week YMCA Graduate Program

A. Warm-up   *10 minutes*
Follow the Walking Warm-up and Standing Warm-up sequences given in Chapter 9. These exercises remain standard for preparation of the body at any stage of exercise intensity. To add variety from session to session, look at the group of alternate stretching and limbering-up calisthenics also described in Chapter 9.

B. Muscular Strength and Flexibility 14 minutes
1. *Alternate Knee-Bend Kicks*
   (page 133)   *20 times*
2. *Regular Lateral Leg Raises, Right   10 times*
   Take same position as in Short Leg Raise (page 133): lie on the left side, support head on left elbow and place other hand on hip. Raise the right leg laterally (upward) as high as possible while keeping the knee straight. Lower the leg, but do not allow it to come in contact with the other leg on the down swing. Stretches side muscles of the thighs.
3. *Flutter Kick on Back (page 134) 30 seconds*
4. *Regular Lateral Leg Raises, Left   10 times*
   Same as No. 2 but for left leg.

156

5. *Regular Push-ups (page 141)*   *10 times*
Do not exceed ten push-ups at one time; the exercise is repeated in smaller sets as indicated below.

6. *Regular Sit-ups (page 140)*   *15 times*
Do not overdo the sit-ups, either, but divide into sets as shown here. Also note the deliberate shifts in this sequence from one muscle group to another: e.g., flutter kick between sets of leg raises, and shoulder squeezer between sets of sit-ups and push-ups.

7. *Isometric Shoulder Squeezer*   *6 times*

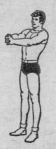

Thrust arms forward and clasp fingers of hands as shown, keeping elbows at shoulder level. Extend upper arms to sides, allowing elbows to bend, and at the same time pulling shoulder blades together. Hold this isometric contraction (i.e., shoulder blades pulling against hands) for six counts. Allow arms and shoulders to relax before repeating exercise. For back muscles.

8. *Sit-ups, second set*   *6 times*
9. *Push-ups, second set*   *6 times*
The next three stretching exercises for muscles of the lower limbs are intended as preparation for jogging, that is, for the cardiovascular training segment that follows.

10. *Thigh Stretcher (page 137)*   *3 left, 3 right*
11. *Hamstring and Calf Stretcher*
    (page 128)   *3 left, 3 right*

12. **Thigh and Leg Stretcher**
    (pages 127-128)   *3 left, 3 right*
13. **Bench Step-ups**   *10 times*

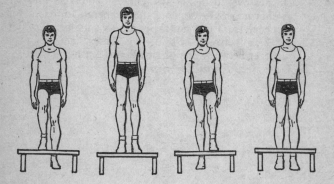

Use a 12-inch-high bench or stair-steps as in the physical fitness test described on page 100. Step up with the right foot; bring up the left foot; step down with the right foot; bring down the left foot. Repeat five times. Then reverse the sequence by starting with the *left* foot; repeat five times. It is necessary to change the sequence so that the same leg does not always bear the burden of lifting and lowering the body. Though the exercise has some cardiovascular value, it is primarily intended here for conditioning muscles of the calves, thighs, and buttocks.

C. *Cardiovascular Training*   *15 minutes*
    1. *Main Street Stroll (page 119)*   *30 seconds*
    2. *Jog (at pace of 10 minutes per*
        mile)   *8 minutes*
    3. *Main Street Stroll (recovery from*
        jog)   *20 seconds*
    4. *Hands Together Overhead*
        (page 147)   *20 seconds*
    5. *Walk with a Twist (page 121)*   *20 seconds*
    6. *Repeat Nos. 3, 4, and 5*   *60 seconds*

WEEKLY PROGRESSIONS FOR INTERMEDIATES

Week	Warm-up (min.)	Muscular Strength & Endurance				C. V. Training			Cool-off (min.)	Total Time (min.)
		Sit-ups	Push-ups	Step-ups	Time (min.)	Jog (min.)	Walk (min.)	Repetitions		
11	10	6	6	10	14	8 1½	2 1	1 3	5	45
12	10	7	6	10	13	9 2	2 1	1 2	5	45
13	10	8	7	15	13	10 2½	2 1	1 2	5	45
14	10	9	7	15	12	11 5	2 2	1 1	5	45
15	10	10	8	20	12	7	2	2	5	45
16	10	11	8	20	12	8	2	2	5	45
17	10	12	9	25	11	9	2	2	5	45
18	10	13	9	25	11	10	2	2	5	45
19	10	14	10	25	10	10	2	2	5	45
20	10	15	10	25	10	10 (2 miles)	—	1	5	45

7. *Jog*	*90 seconds*
8. *Repeat Nos. 3, 4, and 5*	*60 seconds*
9. *Jog*	*90 seconds*
10. *Repeat Nos. 3, 4, and 5*	*60 seconds*
11. *Jog*	*90 seconds*
12. *Repeat Nos. 3, 4, and 5*	*60 seconds*

The jogging sets and timing here are as specified for the first week of the intermediate program. The time given to continuous jogging progressively increases over the ten weeks see the chart on page 159.

D. *Cool-down*

Follow the same pattern of mingling periods of walking and slow jogging as in the beginner's program (page 149), but reduce the total time for cool-down to about five minutes. This can be done simply by cutting the last repetition of the exercises on page 148 (Nos. 1–4, Main Street Stroll, Forward Crawl Stroke, etc). Gradually bring your walk to a halt.

At this point, take your pulse. If the heart rate has not recovered to 100 beats per minute or less, continue walking for another two or three laps. Ordinarily, after ten weeks of conditioning in the beginner's program, your body will need less time for recovery.

As a variation, insert some stretching exercises (page 124) or the Upside-Down Bicycle (page 161) after the last jog. They help not only to cool down in general, but to relieve any muscular tension or soreness that may result from heavy jogging.

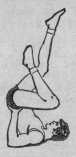

Lie on floor with hips supported by hands as shown. Make pedaling motion with legs as if riding a bicycle, or make a number of scissoring motions, or both. Perform at slow to moderate pace—an ideal exercise for part of the cooling-off period following intensive exercise.

Weekly Schedule for Intermediates

The chart on page 159 gives the exercise schedule and timing for the second, intermediate ten weeks. Note that in the muscular strength and flexibility segment, the number of repetitions increases each week for push-ups, sit-ups, and step-ups. Repetitions of other exercises, listed earlier in this chapter but not included in the weekly chart, may remain constant. Abdominal and upper body development is emphasized in the YMCA selection of calisthenics; the jogging provides exercise for the lower body.

You can vary the number of repetitions or the selection of exercises more or less ad lib, so long as you do not drop below the minimum specified in either the weekly progression chart or in the model program. Analyze your progress constantly to determine what you might need. For example, if you experience muscle soreness after jogging, you should shift the calisthenic emphasis for a while to leg and thigh stretching.

The recovery intervals after each period of jogging offer another variable; you may need more or less time for recovery as determined by your pulse rate. The walking times specified in the chart are calculated to hold the total workout time within forty to forty-five minutes.

Ready for the Ski Slope?

It has been mentioned in this book that systematic exercise provides a valuable *preparation* for sports: that you should not depend on weekly sets of tennis, weekend skiing, etc., to improve or maintain your physical fitness. On the contrary, some sports can be anti-fitness in the sense of leading to muscular accidents: strains, sprains, or even broken bones. A fit person makes a better player because he can "take it." He can muster the extra energy for that winning point without getting hurt.

Skiing is a case typical of many modern sports. In its beginnings, the ski slope was a place only for physically rugged young men. They had to climb a mountain on foot before they could come sliding down it on skis. One of the early ski centers in this country, Tuckerman's Ravine on the slope of Mt. Washington, N.H., won its following because unusually good hiking trails passable in almost any weather brought the skier to the head of a snowbound ravine at about 4,000 feet altitude.

Ski lifts, comfortable lodgings, motor roads, and other "civilized" amenities have taken practically all of the toughness out of recreational skiing, while artificial hills and machine-made snow have spread the sport to the undemanding lowlands. Hence, skiing every year attracts unsuspecting people out for fun with little or no realization of the physical demands upon them. The ski beginner's broken leg has become a cartoon cliché.

A good skier must have:

• *Endurance*—the stamina to finish one run and be ready for the next one; to keep going when the going is rough; to withstand bad weather; or to meet the unexpected situation without undue fatigue.

• *Strength and power*—the ability to stand firm on his skis and control their direction and to make his way cross country or uphill as necessary.

- *Flexibility*—the ability to bounce up from an impact or upset and to recover quickly.
- *Agility* in making a wide range of motions and in changing motion instantly and accurately.
- *Coordination* of muscular movements and the ability to concentrate.
- *Relaxation*—the power to relax from tension and thus avoid stiffness or awkwardness in movement.

Those are the elements of a YMCA physical fitness program designed for skiers, whether beginners or experts. It is aimed at enabling the individual to participate successfully, enjoyably, *and safely*. It should begin several weeks before the season starts.

The program here may also be adapted to other sports; after all, a skier's fitness needs are not basically different from those of any sports enthusiast who wants to play hard but not suffer injury.

The YMCA Preskiing Program

The program is divided into three fitness phases: beginning, intermediate, and advanced. The content remains the same throughout, but increases in intensity as measured by the number of repetitions of an exercise or in the time devoted to it. Place yourself in the appropriate class *not* according to your skiing skill but according to your ability to complete the beginner's or intermediate exercise sequences given earlier in this book.

1. Run or jog the distance indicated at right. Make note of your time, which should equal the "graduate" beginner's rate of one mile in ten minutes.	Beg. ½ mile Int. 1 mile Adv. 1 mile

2. Chair Step-ups

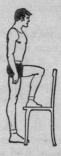

Stand facing a chair. Step up onto the chair leading with left foot. Bring up right foot and stand on chair. Step down with left foot.
Beg. 25 times
Int. 50 times
Adv. 100 times

Step down with right foot. Do half of the repetitions in this sequence; then lead with the right foot for the remaining repetitions.

3. Side-to-Side Jumping

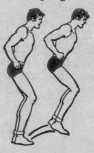

Stand with feet and knees together, knees bent. Jump at least two feet from left to right, then back from right to left in each repetition.
Beg. 10 times
Int. 20 times
Adv. 30 times

4. Burpee (for men)

Squat down, placing hands in front of feet. Put weight on hands, but keep arms straight. Thrust both legs backward so that you support

Beg. 5 times
Int. 10 times
Adv. 15 times

yourself on hands and feet. Then bend arms but keep body straight until chest touches floor between your hands. Push body up. Bring both feet together back to kneeling position. Stand up; then repeat exercise.

Burpee (for women)

The complete Burpee for men is a six-count exercise; women should do only four counts, omitting the push-up portion; that is, (1) squat; (2) kick feet forward; (3) kick feet back again; (4) stand erect.

5. Knee-to-Shoulder Hop

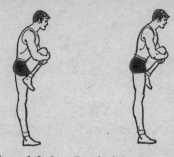

Stand on left leg. Bend right leg
and pull up knee with hands as if
trying to place it against your right
shoulder. Then start rhythmically

Beg. 10 times
Int. 20 times
Adv. 30 times

hopping from left leg to right leg, exchanging knees.
Bringing both knees in turn up to the shoulder equals
one repetition.

6. Curling Sit-up

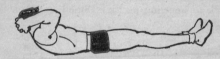

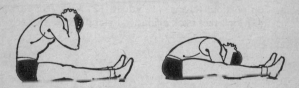

Lie on back with legs apart, knees
bent, and feet flat on floor. Join
hands behind neck or extend them
straight out behind you. Raise the

Beg. 5 times
Int. 10 times
Adv. 20 times

head by placing the chin on the chest and rounding
the shoulders. Curl up to a sitting position. Continue
bending from hips until head is between the knees.
Return to starting position and repeat.

Guidelines for Skiers

As stated earlier, the main elements of physical fitness for skiing are endurance; strength and power; flexibility; agility; coordination; and relaxation. Therefore, a daily conditioning program should include exercises that strengthen, stretch, and relax the muscles of the arms, shoulders, abdomen, back, and legs. It should also give the heart and lungs a vigorous workout.

Exercising should not reach the point of exhaustion, but it is suggested to repeat each exercise one or two times more than you feel you can do at the moment. The training effect will depend upon a continuous increase in the work load, whether measured by the duration, number of repetitions, or difficulty of the exercising.

After a strenuous exercise, relax! Do an easier exercise or a few breathing exercises. Work variety into your program. While running, alternate between jogging and short all-out wind sprints.

Try to complete the above workout at least three times a week. If the workout takes you less than fifteen minutes, move up to the intermediate level. If the advanced level is too hard for you, just stay at the intermediate level for a while. You can't become fit overnight, especially after a long layoff. Work up slowly to a harder workout, and press yourself at least a little to improve.

This will be true even if you are an "advanced" or expert skier. Skill depends upon knowledge and practice, but your ability to put that skill into practice on the ski slopes and trails depends on your condition—the ability of your muscles, nerves, and vital organs to meet the challenge.

Introduction to Jogging

Jogging is a sport as well as an exercise, and a sociable sport which can include an entire family, neighborhood, club, church group, etc. The popularity of jogging rallies and competitive runs such as the Boston Marathon seems to increase every year. Like any other sport, jogging is only for people in fit condition—but the jogging itself may be programmed to help you attain that condition.

The YMCA jogging program is introductory, aimed to develop the individual's ability to run. The overload principle may be applied either by increasing the distance or the speed. When the distance is limited by time, then the overload must be obtained by running faster.

Note that jogging and running are the same thing physiologically, though in popular usage jogging is a relatively slow run, while running may be at a sprinter's pace. Usually a training stimulus in jogging is attained with the heart rate above 135 beats per minute.

Persons over 50 years of age, individuals who are in very poor condition, and the obese should start with the walking program (Chapter 12) and postpone intensive jogging until they have attained a fair level of fitness by walking. On the other hand, experienced or well-conditioned runners can start at a higher level than the introductory program in this chapter, since they are able to work and progress much faster.

Although jogging is primarily a leg exercise, it is important to strengthen the musculature of the abdomen, shoulder girdle, and back. A jogger should include at least three warm-up and stretching calisthenics in each workout.

YMCA Jogging Program

The YMCA schedule for joggers has three divisions: (1) a preconditioning or pretraining period of three weeks, during which some muscle soreness and stiffness can be expected; (2) a conditioning period of five weeks; and (3) the running program proper, for full-fledged joggers able to cover at least six miles per week. During the first two periods, a *daily* workout is suggested; after that, try to work out as many times as possible, no less than twice a week.

Preconditioning Period

First week daily schedule
1. Warm up by stretching, twisting, bending exercises (Chapter 9). Concentrate on muscles in the back of the legs and the inside of the thighs.
2. Walk 200 yards.
3. Touch toes, stretch legs, twist at waist, circle arms (Chapter 10).

4. Jog 50 yards, walk 50 yards, and repeat for a total of 6 times.
5. Rest for two minutes.
6. Do push-ups, sit-ups (Chapter 10), and chest raising.

Chest Raising

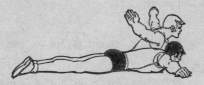

Lie on front with hands clasped behind head and feet held down by a partner. Slowly and carefully, raise head and chest off floor. Return to original position and repeat.

7. Walk 100 yards, jog 100 yards, and repeat for a total of four times.

Second Week
1–3. Same as first week.
4. Jog 50 yards, walk 50 yards, 8 repetitions.
5, 6. Same as first week.
7. Jog 100 yards, walk 100 yards, 6 repetitions.

Third Week
1–3. Same as first week.
4. Jog 50 yards, walk 50 yards, 8 repetitions.
5, 6. Same as first week.
7. Jog 100 yards, walk 100 yards, 10 repetitions.

Conditioning Period

Fourth Week
First 3 days:
1. Warm up.
2. Run 100 yards, walk 100 yards, 5 repetitions.

3. Rest and calisthenics as in previous weeks.
4. Run 50 yards, walk 100 yards, 5 repetitions.

4th and 5th days:
1. Warm up.
2. Run 100 yards, walk 100 yards, 9 repetitions.
3. Rest and calisthenics.
4. Run 200 yards.

Fifth Week
Same as preceding, except at No. 4, run 300 yards.

Sixth Week
Same as preceding, except at No. 4, run 400 yards.

Seventh Week
1. Warm up.
2. Run 100 yards, walk 50 yards, 12 repetitions.
3. Rest and calisthenics.
4. Run 500 yards.

Eighth Week
1. Warm up.
2. Run 150 yards, walk 50 yards, 9 repetitions.
3. Rest and calisthenics.
4. Run 600 yards.

Running Period

Ninth Week and succeeding weeks
Increase running and reduce walking, for combined total of six miles per week. Be sure always to warm up before each workout.

If competitive running is planned, training should be steadily increased in severity, but only after an extensive physical examination by an M.D. When preparing for a race, include heat adaptation by training on hot days and with the sun high. The added stress of competition thus will be physiologically expected.

A competitive run should not be the runner's first exposure to stress or to heat. Don't allow team pressure or social pressure to push you beyond your normal limits.

Chapter 12

WALKING, CYCLING, AND SWIMMING

Thus far in this book, we have had in mind the typical case of a person who is (a) in poor *physical* condition, needing remedial exercise, but (b) in reasonably good *medical* condition, able to tolerate exercise. This person should be able to undergo a ten-week beginner's program of progressive exercise intensity and to emerge in an improved state of fitness ready for almost anything—a couple of fast sets of tennis or a high peak in Colorado, or a more strenuous exercise program to hone his body conditioning to an athlete's sharpness.

Some people for one reason or another can't fit these typical criteria. They need systematic preparation even before beginning a "beginner's" program. To put it on a personal level, even if you could not pass the physical fitness tests described in Chapter 8, you are by no means "out of it." There is still a place for you on the exercise scene.

Practically everyone can walk. Even a recent cardiac patient fresh out of hospital can and should walk for exercise. And simply by walking on a scientific schedule, our out-of-shape prebeginner, our "freshman," can achieve a very satisfactory, rewarding training effect and better health.

At a YMCA, when a person's measured level of cardiovascular output is too low to attempt a jogging program, the member is switched to the walking program. Potential candidates include:

- Anyone over 60 years old.
- Anyone scoring poorly on cardiovascular fitness tests.
- Anyone with high blood pressure.
- Anyone who is overweight to the point of obesity.

171

- Anyone with orthopedic problems or other conditions of the joints, bones, etc., that make calisthenics difficult or impossible.

Happily, the walking program offers a worthy alternative to jogging as a cardiovascular endurance workout. The purpose is to develop a level of fitness high enough to enter the beginner's exercise program. This progress is achieved in exactly the same way as described in other programs in this book—by gradually increasing the work load as the body adjusts to greater and greater energy output.

Guidelines for a Walker

The YMCA program schedules ten weeks of walking a distance that gradually increases and at a pace set by the clock. The ultimate objective is sufficient fitness to walk two miles in thirty minutes, that is, at an average speed of four miles per hour. The selected speed is calculated to increase the walker's energy expenditure four to six times the basal metabolic rate. In short, the result is the same as from a very good calisthenic or jogging workout, although spread over a longer period of time.

Programmed walking is done at two different paces. The *endurance pace* equals four miles per hour, the pace of the program's two-mile objective. The *alternating pace* consists of alternately walking at four miles per hour for *no more than four minutes* followed by a period of slower, leisurely walking. The principle of the alternating pace is exactly the same as in the jog-walk-jog sequence of a jogging program, but applied at a lower level of intensity. The progressive time intervals are listed in the weekly schedule that follows.

If you find the scheduled pace too fast, do not be concerned; simply walk slower. But *cover the entire distance* even if it takes you half a day. Eventually your condition will improve so that you can cover the distance faster; you will see the improvement reflected in pulse rates.

Remember that the time goals for walking are not a bus schedule; you can miss a connection here and there without harm. Absolutely strict adherence to the recommended walking pace is not necessary, but it *is* important to evince an exercise response.

In most people, the endurance pace should induce a heart

rate of 120–130 beats per minute—but not more. Take your pulse often and watch out for overstress. The pulse rate should drop below 120 beats per minute within three minutes after the exertion.

Warm up before walking. This may seem like a contradiction, since walking itself is a warm-up exercise in the programs previously described. But believe it or not, the kind of fast walking prescribed here can be heavy work for the unfit. It will subject your circulatory system as well as certain muscles to real training stress. Before setting out on a fast stroll, devote five minutes or so to advance warm-up and stretching exercises—such as those in Chapter 9.

The YMCA Walking Schedule

The progression schedule calls for three walks a week for ten weeks. On intervening days do as much "ordinary" walking as you can manage—for instance by leaving the car at home and running errands on foot. *Continuity* and *regularity* are essential; the walks are adding fitness a little at a time and you want the effect to be cumulative. Set up your program for three days a week and keep the dates without fail, rain or shine.

Walking is more readily timed and measured in a gymnasium or on an outdoor track, but of course you can ambulate in any kind of territory. Simply try to find some place with minimum interruptions. Avoid busy streets and heavy traffic. If you have to stop at every corner to wait for the light, the training effect you want from walking will be inhibited.

In the following recommended series of walks, each week sets up a new distance or a new time goal, or both; and each day specifies the period at the endurance pace and the period at the alternating pace. These are geared to the time you will need for recovery, in the expectation that you'll develop more and more endurance and need less and less recovery time as you go along.

The schedule assumes that you will complete the entire warm-up routine (Chapter 9) before starting each day's walk.

First Week—Distance ¾ mile; time goal 12 minutes.
 Day 1—Alternating pace; endurance rate (i.e., 4 mph) should be used up to half of the time.

Day 2—Alternating pace; endurance rate up to three-fourths of the time.

Day 3—Endurance pace; aim for ¾ mile in 12 minutes.

Second week—Distance 1 mile; time goal 15 minutes.

Day 1—Endurance pace—½ mile; alternating pace—½ mile.

Day 2—Endurance pace—¾ mile; alternating pace—¼ mile.

Day 3—Endurance pace—1 mile; aim for 1 mile in 15 minutes.

Third Week—Distance 1¼ miles; time goal 19 minutes.

Day 1—Endurance pace—½ mile; alternating pace—¾ mile.

Day 2—Endurance pace—¾ mile; alternating pace—½ mile.

Day 3—Repeat.

Fourth week—Distance 1¼ miles; time goal 19 minutes.

Day 1—Endurance pace—1 mile; alternating pace—¼ mile.

Day 2—Repeat.

Day 3—Endurance pace—1¼ miles; aim for time goal of 19 minutes.

Fifth week—Distance 1½ miles; time goal 23 minutes.

Day 1—Endurance pace—¾ mile; alternating pace—¾ mile.

Day 2—Endurance pace—1 mile; alternating pace—½ mile.

Day 3—Repeat.

Sixth week—Distance 1½ miles; time goal 23 minutes.

Day 1—Endurance pace—1¼ miles; alternating pace—¼ mile.

Day 2—Repeat.

Day 3—Endurance pace—aim for time goal of 23 minutes.

Seventh week—Distance 1¾ miles; time goal 26 minutes.

Day 1—Endurance pace—1 mile; alternating pace—¾ mile.

Day 2—Endurance pace—1¼ miles; alternating pace—½ mile.

Day 3—Repeat.

Eighth week—Distance 1¾ miles; time goal 26 minutes.
  Day 1—Endurance pace—1½ miles; alternating pace—¼ mile.
  Day 2—Repeat.
  Day 3—Endurance pace—1¾ miles; aim for time goal of 26 minutes.

Ninth week—Distance 2 miles; time goal 30 minutes.
  Day 1—Endurance pace—1¼ miles; alternating pace—¾ mile.
  Day 2—Endurance pace—1½ miles; alternating pace—½ mile.
  Day 3—Repeat.

Tenth week—Distance 2 miles; time goal 30 minutes.
  Day 1—Endurance pace—1¾ miles; alternating pace—¼ mile.
  Day 2—Repeat.
  Day 3—Endurance pace 2 miles; aim at time goal of 30 minutes.

The walking program can be based on time instead of distance if convenient. This might prove advantageous in a scenic outdoor area or in a gymnasium not marked for distance. Suitable progressive time intervals are shown in the table below.

WALKING PROGRAM—TIME INTERVALS
(in minutes)

Week	Day 1 End. Pace	Day 1 Alt. Pace	Day 2 End. Pace	Day 2 Alt. Pace	Day 3 End. Pace	Day 3 Alt. Pace	Total Time (min.)
1		12		12	12		12
2	7½	7½	12	3	15		15
3	10	9	14	5	14	5	19
4	15	4	15	4	19		19
5	12	11	15	8	15	8	23
6	18	5	18	5	23		23
7	15	11	19	7	19	7	26
8	22	4	22	4	26		26
9	19	11	23	7	23	7	30
10	26	4	26	4	30		30

Training on the Bicycle Ergometer

A stationary bicycle like the one aboard the Skylab spaceship or used in physical fitness testing offers a very convenient way of setting up a program of controlled exercise. The machine is compact. Most gymnasiums own at least one, and many people have one installed at home. Regulating the work load is simple and accurate.

Training on a bicycle ergometer is particularly suitable for the prebeginner or "freshman" who temporarily can't quite make the grade in a regular course of body conditioning.

The apparatus is called an ergometer because a measurable work load (in ergs) can be readily applied, and adjusted according to the need. Usually this is done by imposing a resistance or brake against the rider's pedaling, set to measure on a graduated scale. At *zero* on the scale there is no resistance and the bicycle wheel turns freely. At *seven,* the highest setting on most ergometers, the wheel won't turn without very vigorous pumping.

The bicycle ergometer is a good substitute for jogging when people have a low score in the cardiovascular fitness test. It is suitable for the obese and those with leg soreness or other conditions that make running difficult, if not impossible. Cycling may occasionally substitute for jogging by a physically fit person, say on a rainy day.

Guidelines for Cycling

The rider performs continuously at a tempo which elicits a heart rate response equal to 60 to 80 percent of the maximum for his age. The load on the machine starts at zero and is gradually increased until the desired heart rate as calculated is attained. The ride continues for a specified period of time. As physical condition improves over the weeks or months, the intensity of the exercise is increased. The intensity should be constantly evaluated and regulated according to the following recommended procedure:

1. On the first day, ride the bicycle at 50 revolutions per minute with zero load for two minutes.

2. Increase the load to 150 kilograms per minute (kpm), maintain the 50 rpm pedaling rate, and continue for two more minutes.

3. Just before the two minutes are up, take your pulse. If the heart rate has not reached the desired range (see below), increase the work load another 150 kpm.

Desired range: The exercise heart rate (EHR) is a percentage from 60 to 80 of the maximum heart rate (MHR) determined by age. An approximate MHR equals 220 minus the person's age. The low end of the 60-to-80 percentage scale is observed for the very unfit person; the upper end for persons with some degree of body conditioning already attained. For example, assume a person 50 years old, who is very sedentary and just starting to exercise:

$$MHR = 220 - 50 = 170 \text{ beats per minute}$$
$$EHR = .60 \times 170 = 102 \text{ beats per minute}$$

The heart rate during the exercise should keep within 5 beats per minute of the EHR, that is, the desired range is from 97 to 107 beats per minute in the above example.

4. Continue increasing the load 150 kilograms at a time while checking the heart rate (i.e., repeat steps 2 and 3) until the EHR does fall within the desired range as calculated.

5. When the heart rate comes within range, continue pedaling for eight *more* minutes (ten minutes altogether at this load). Check the pulse from time to time to make sure the heart is not accelerating out of range. Adjust the work load downward if it is. This procedure will establish a correct work load to apply in bicycle exercising for one week.

6. When the ten minutes are up, reduce the load by 150 kpm at one-minute intervals until zero load is reached. Continue riding at zero load until you feel like coming to a stop, usually in one and a half or two minutes. DO NOT STOP PEDALING SUDDENLY. As in any other exercise, you need a cool-down; and in this case, a careful tapering off is absolutely essential to prevent blood pooling in the lower limbs.

7. On subsequent days, always start at zero load and work up; always taper off by working the load back down in steps to zero.

8. At the beginning of the next week, evaluate the heart rate response again. If it still equals the desired percent of MHR (60 percent in our example), use the same work load

for another week. If the heart rate is less than desired, increase the load in the same manner as in steps 1–4 above.

9. As the weeks pass and physical condition improves, the relative intensity of the exercise can be increased by upping the percentage factor in the heart rate equation. Thus, in the case of our 50-year-old sedentary man, the EHR may be increased from 60 percent of MHR to 70 percent, if at the former level there appears to be relatively little real exertion.

It is desirable to use 70 to 80 percent as a regular training stimulus once it has become established that the rider tolerates the exercise well and shows no signs of overstrain. A well-conditioned person using the bicycle as a temporary alternative to jogging can safely start at the 70–80 percent level.

Note: If no training effect appears at the beginning of the program—if the load does *not* have to be increased to elicit the desired heart rate response—you should see a doctor. There is a good chance some medical problem exists that causes a rapid heart beat independently of exercise.

Road Bicycles

Riding a bicycle as a vehicle of transportation is good cardiovascular endurance exercise, somewhat more intensive than fast walking. However, employing road cycling for a controlled exercise program presents difficulties because there are many different kinds of bicycles and all kinds of roads. The invention of the 3-speed and then the 10-speed bike created the bicycle boom of recent years by enabling a rider to pedal up grades without dismounting.

Middle-aged people who try to ride a bicycle for the first time since childhood often are astounded at how arduous it seems. For them, a program of stationary bicycling would provide fine preparation in the form of cardiovascular and muscular conditioning.

In a 10-speed bike, the tenth speed is the lowest gear, giving the rider the greatest mechanical advantage. Ninth speed gives him a little less mechanical advantage, eighth speed still less, and so on. This suggests a way to gradually increase a bicycling work load to achieve a training effect.

The rider selects a stretch of road with a steep grade he can easily climb in tenth gear. He does this for a few days. Then he tackles the same grade in ninth gear; he keeps at it until the hill presents no difficulties. Next he shifts to eighth gear for the same grade. He keeps lowering the gear ratio until finally he reaches a gear, say the third or fourth, in which he can't overcome the grade but must get off and walk his bike up the hill. He shifts to the next lower gear and continues riding with that load.

In ordinary bicycle cruising, the amount of exercise involved may be related to the 10-minute-mile of jogging, which is the training objective of the YMCA beginner's program. According to the aerobic charts of Dr. K. H. Cooper, the equivalent training effect on a bicycle would be achieved by riding three miles in nine minutes. The jogger in the intermediate program does two miles in twenty minutes; the equivalent on a bike would be about five and a half miles in twenty minutes.

These equivalents are very rough approximations for general guidance only. They assume a cycling course with equal time uphill and downhill, also equal time with the wind and against the wind. Since a bike in high gear can go much faster than the 18–20 mph indicated by the equivalents, maintaining this *average* speed might involve some faster spurts with periods of less intensive cruising in between.

The 50-Mile Swim

Swimming ranks with walking as virtually an ideal exercise for the physically unfit starting on their way back to endurance, health, and agility. Depending on the tempo and the stroke used, a swim can be restful and relaxing or it can be strenuous in the extreme. Vigorous swimming develops all-round strength and endurance, especially when several different strokes are employed to involve different muscles and when the distances swum are progressively increased.

Since the pace of swimming is self-limiting—you can't go any faster or any longer than your heart and lungs will permit —the dangers of overstress are minimal in the confines of a swimming pool. A training effect is achieved in the water simply by repetition. In many YMCA's the program is called a 50-Mile Swim.

That distance—50 miles—seems enormous, unattainable. It is about twice the distance across the English Channel that won fame for swimmer Gertrude Ederle and others. Many would find a mere 200 yards tough going and would be proud to cover that distance in six minutes or less. But remember, you can visualize 50 miles merely as the sum of a lot of 200-yard or even 100-yard swims. If you swim a given distance each day you will eventually attain 50 miles—and here's the point:

A training effect in swimming as in walking is *cumulative*. You will keep improving in physical fitness so long as you continue swimming regularly, or at least until your body reaches a steady state of output matching your age and physical structure. Consequently, to set up a 50-mile swim program is a matter of simple arithmetic.

Guidelines for Pool Swimming

1. Determine the length of the swimming pool, and the number of days each week that it will be available.

2. Set a time limit on completing your 50 miles. Six months is a typical choice for beginners.

3. Multiply 26 weeks (six months) by the number of days each week that you will be swimming. This gives the number of swimming sessions in your schedule. For instance, if you use the pool five times a week, you will have $5 \times 26 = 130$ swimming sessions all told.

4. Convert 50 miles into yards and divide by the number of sessions. The result is the distance you will have to *average* per swim to complete the program. For example:

$$50 \text{ miles} = 50 \times 1{,}760 \text{ yards} = 88{,}000 \text{ yards.}$$
$$\frac{88{,}000 \text{ yards}}{130 \text{ sessions}} = 677 \text{ yards per session} = \text{⅜ of a mile (approx.)}$$

5. Divide this average distance by the lap length of the pool. The result is the *number of laps* you must swim at each session *on the average*.

When swimming pools at YMCA's, high schools, etc., are also used for competitive events, lap lengths are generally divisible into a standard distance such as 220 yards or the equivalent metric distance. E.g., in a 66-foot pool (equals 22 yards), there would be exactly 10 laps to 220 yards, or 80 laps to the mile.

6. Having done the arithmetic, now look at the problem in physical terms. A middle-aged person in flabby condition, just beginning to exercise, may be unable to swim anywhere near three-eighths of a mile without frequent rests. He would be winded probably within one-eighth of a mile, or even less, if he tried to swim continuously.

Hence, on the first day, swim only as many laps as you can without suffering distress—and then swim a couple of laps more. On the second day, try to swim a little farther; on the third day, still farther; and so on until you have attained the average number of laps required by your 50-mile program. You will find the goal easier to reach each day.

7. Swim the average number of laps for a week or longer. Then progressively increase the distance a lap or two each day. Remember that you will have to exceed the average distance during the later weeks of the 50-mile program in order to make up for deficiencies during the early weeks. As time passes, you will find this presents no difficulty.

Note: If this regimen seems too strenuous, simply lengthen the time period for the 50-mile swim to nine months, ten months, or even longer. The Red Cross awards a badge for 50 miles in three *years*.

Swimming Definitions

In swimming for exercise you are not in a race. If you can't swim continuously for more than a few laps, simply take longer about it *but keep moving*. Switch from crawl stroke to breast stroke and back; tread water; puff and blow to catch your breath.

Don't worry about overstrain—practically impossible in a swimming pool unless perhaps under the great emotional pressure of saving someone from drowning. Most water accidents occur at a beach from swimming too far from shore and then panicking at the effort of getting back. In a pool they may be caused by collisions or inexpert diving—not exhaustion.

The relative strenuousness of different swimming strokes is indicated by the following table of energy output.

SWIMMING ENERGY OUTPUT (*Dependent on Speed*)
(*in calories per minute*)

Breast stroke	7.0
Backstroke	8.0
Crawl stroke	9.0
Butterfly stroke	12.0

Using the jogging standard of one mile in ten minutes for comparison, a crawl stroke swim of a quarter mile (440 yards) in ten minutes would produce approximately the equivalent training effect. The butterfly stroke would produce the same effect in a shorter distance; the backstroke and breast stroke would take longer.

Swimming is unusual among forms of exercise in being performed with the body held horizontally, as if on all fours. For this reason it encourages correct positioning and adjustment of vertebrae and joints. Swimming is often recommended for persons having lower back pain or other musculoskeletal problems occasioned or exacerbated by the upright posture. President F. D. Roosevelt popularized swimming as an exercise for people who, like himself, had been crippled by polio.

Aquatics are a relatively painless way to get a good workout for the heart and circulatory system.

Chapter 13

THE "Y" WAY OF LIFE

The down-pointed equilateral triangle of the YMCA represents the three sides of a balanced personality: body, mind, and at the top, spirit. The symbol was originated in 1890 by Dr. Luther H. Gulick, the organization's first national secretary for physical education, with this explanation:

"Man is essentially a unity: body, mind, and spirit, each being a necessary and eternal part of man, he being neither one alone but all three . . . each contributing a proportionate development of man's whole nature."

The concept of the "whole man," involving not only his physical health and his mental powers but his spiritual stability and religious attitudes, is the unique contribution of the YMCA to the modern pursuit of physical fitness. It says in effect that the body, as a gift of God, imposes a personal responsibility upon the individual, in his mind and spirit, to take as good care of it as possible.

The Young Men's Christian Association began in London, England, in 1844 as a spontaneous uplift movement for "the improvement of the spiritual and mental condition of commercial young men." A young draper's assistant named George Williams became disenchanted with the dreary existence of young bachelors in the ugly new world of the industrial revolution. He organized a small group of his fellow dry goods clerks to meet regularly for Bible readings, "mental culture," and fellowship—in other words, to have a little fun together without getting drunk and disorderly.

It was an idea whose time had come. It spread rapidly among the employees of business firms in London and received some publicity in religious journals. In 1851, it crossed the Atlantic Ocean to Boston, Massachusetts, where Thomas V. Sullivan, a retired sea captain imbued with missionary zeal, established the first American YMCA. That English seed grew lushly on American soil. By 1860, there were said to be 205 YMCA's with 25,000 members in cities throughout the United States.

At first, the chief concern of the association leaders was to look after country youths first arriving in the peril-strewn city. Revival meetings, street corner sermons, and distribution of tracts by "gospel wagons" featured their work. Then came the Civil War, which broadened the rather narrow original concept and made the "Y" famous. It abandoned sectarianism and became eclectic, open to all who accepted its general purposes.

During the war some 5,000 men and women from YMCA's became volunteer workers, serving the personal needs of the troops from hot coffee to letters home—the first volunteer agency for spiritual and physical aid to American armed forces. They did not cringe from the front lines; they were officially commended by President Lincoln. Forty men and three women lost their lives in this service.

Birth of Physical Education

As early as 1856, groups within the YMCA had begun advocating that since "bodily health is intimately connected with mental and spiritual activity and development," the associations should provide "properly conducted" gymnasiums and baths. The first breakthrough came in 1858, when the Brooklyn, N.Y., association installed bowling alleys, excusing its daring action with the statement: "The amusement question must be faced; men whose principal occupation is brain work need muscular amusement."

In 1860, the National Convention of the YMCA adopted a resolution favoring the establishment of gymnasiums "as a safeguard against the allurements of objectionable places of resort, which have proved the ruin of thousands of the youth of our country."

The first gym appeared in 1869 as the "physical department" of the new 23rd Street YMCA in New York, planned by pioneer enthusiast Robert R. McBurney and since named after him. The first "swimming bath" or pool was installed at a Brooklyn branch in 1885; it was 45 feet long.

Over the next 20 years it could be said that the YMCA

made athletics respectable. Although three "ivy" colleges, Amherst, Harvard, and Yale, already had gymnasiums, the public or commercial gyms of the time were hangouts for street corner toughs and the "fight game." A minister wrote in 1885:

"The gymnasium used to be a wicked place, a place for pugilists to get a muscle, a training school for manufacturing hoodlums. Now what do you see there? College professors swinging dumbbells, millionaires turning somersaults, lawyers hanging upside down, doctors of divinity punching a bag, dyspeptics on a rope ladder, old age dancing itself young!"

Some of the Pioneers

An earnest young enthusiast for body building, Robert J. Roberts, became physical director of the Boston YMCA in 1877, and in eight years increased its membership from 226 to 1,270. Summing up his contribution, Dr. Gulick wrote:

"[Roberts] developed a distinctive style of gymnastic work which is exceedingly simple, is attractive, can be operated in large classes, is effective in relation to the vital functions of digestion, circulation, and respiration, and which can be successfully taught by teachers of mediocre ability. . . . Among other inventions and improvements we owe to him the indoor shot, the medicine ball, the thick felt mattress, and the felt and canvas running track."

Nevertheless the spread of "physical work," as it was called, met with opposition for about 15 years from religious leaders of the association who could see no relationship between the spiritual and physical natures of man. Roberts proselytized by giving talks on "scientific body building" at YMCA conventions, at one of which:

"He appeared in a gymnasium costume and began with a fervent and simple prayer for wisdom in what he would say. His own physical development was an exhibition in itself. To illustrate his remarks he conducted a class dumbbell drill upon the stage, using eight YMCA secretaries. He also demonstrated feats of strength by himself. His program was enthusiastically applauded."

Springfield College

In 1887, a Department of Physical Training was set up at Springfield (Mass.) College by Luther H. Gulick, the Honolulu-born son of a medical missionary. Gulick had been handicapped in his boyhood by recurrent headaches and uncertain health. As a student at Oberlin College he developed an intense interest in physical education, and after graduation set out for a degree in medicine. Even before he received his M.D. (in 1889), he was deep into revolutionary methods of physical training and education as a dean at Springfield, where the YMCA trained its leaders.

Among other endeavors he established a football team. Its coach was Amos Alonzo Stagg, former theological student at Yale and an All-American football player, later to become one of the most famous of American football coaches. Its star center was James Naismith, a young Canadian divinity student who had played football at McGill. Known as "Stagg's Stubby Christians," the Springfield eleven did pretty well, and after the first year both Stagg and Naismith were appointed to the faculty.

Birth of Basketball

Dean Gulick felt the need of a "new sports game" to re-awaken enthusiasm among Springfield students. Even the revised course of body-building exercises à la Roberts had failed to dispel growing boredom in the gymnasium at Winchester Square. In 1891, Gulick asked Naismith to see what he could do with the class; two teachers had already admitted defeat.

Naismith protested that (a) he knew nothing of gymnastics, and (b) he was already teaching boxing, wrestling, swimming, and canoeing. Gulick suggested that perhaps he could invent a new gymnasium group game to replace some of the calisthenics.

Less than two weeks later, after some heavy thought, a novel concept took shape in Naismith's mind. He lifted one feature from lacrosse, another from rugby football, a third from "duck-on-the-rock." One morning, soccer ball in hand, Naismith poked around in the school basement looking for wooden boxes. He found none, but did locate two old peach baskets. He knocked the bottoms out of the baskets and

186

nailed them, one at each end of the gym, to the lower rail of the balcony. Between them he posted a list of 13 rules. He then "chose up sides" of nine men on each team, tossed them the soccer ball, and told them to see which team could get the ball into its basket most often.

And so basketball was born in a YMCA college gym.

In 1895, another gymnasium game, volleyball, was similarly invented to put fun into exercise by another YMCA training leader, William G. Morgan. Dr. Gulick himself created the pentathlon of five track events, the 100-yard dash, 12-pound hammer throw, running high jump, pole vault, and mile run. We can muse at the astonishment of these pioneers could they see the emergence of basketball as a big-time professional sport, or of "spiking" in modern volleyball and its acceptance as a national subsidized game in such countries as Cuba.

The Way to Well-being

The lesson for us lies in the playing of games at the "Y" for fun and health—not for lucre. In later years the YMCA was to place great emphasis on swimming and life-saving, scuba diving, co-ed work, family work, urban work, and finally physical fitness per se.

The letter "Y" today stands for *sport with social responsibility,* and not only in the original YMCA. Today we have such emulative organizations as the YWCA (Young Women's Christian Association), the CYO (Catholic Youth Organization), and YMWHA (Young Men's and Women's Hebrew Association). The latter was originated as the YMHA in 1874 by Jewish members of the New York YMCA.

In considering the contemporary world of supersonic speed, instant worldwide communication, pressures, tensions, anxieties, and complexity, coupled with too much food, excessive use of alcohol, tobacco, and drugs, and lack of physical activity, we might well ponder the following statement made by Dr. Gulick in 1891:

"Our physical education should be all around; have reference to spiritual and mental growth; be educative and progressive; give each man what he individually needs; and be interesting."

The "Y" Looks Ahead

In the past five years, the YMCA alone has brought the body conditioning and physical fitness message to over 20 million men, women, and children who have participated in its programs. In the next five years, a new YMCA concept now in the planning stage would enlist millions more in a frontal attack on the nation's most devastating single health problem: cardiovascular disease.

The magnitude of the problem, more correctly an epidemic, has been mentioned earlier in this book. If just one day has passed since you read that, 4,000 more Americans have suffered a heart attack—for that is the average number stricken every day. In 1971, 675,000 of the heart attack victims died. In the same year, an estimated 3,800,000 persons had coronary artery disease. Heart trouble and blood circulation trouble—cardiovascular disease—kill more people in the United States than all other causes of death combined.

In its physical fitness programs, such as those described in this book, the YMCA already has placed maximum emphasis on cardiovascular training through exercise. These programs, however, are essentially for healthy (though unfit) individuals. But today it is estimated that one American in every eight—27 million men, women, and even children—suffer from some form of cardiovascular disease, and most of them have not been diagnosed.

To meet this challenge, the YMCA now contemplates created "cardiovascular health centers" and certified fitness activity centers in addition to its present 931 physical education centers. Their functions would be designed specifically to provide a badly needed public service for early detection of cardiovascular disease, as through stress testing; for scientific preventive or rehabilitative measures, as through exercise testing and prescription; and for public education, training, and research in this field. Thus in 1972, the YMCA administered 97,351 physical fitness tests. Under the proposed nationwide program, this could expand to several millions. It would embrace not only the healthy but those in danger of, or having actually suffered, a myocardial infarction.

Action and Effort—Now

If this book has helped you, the reader, to a more positive view of the healthful life, it has served its purpose.

The only sure way to physical well-being does not lie in fads or quickie diets or magic health spa machines or in mystical notions from the ancient East, but in *action and effort* right here and now—to work out regularly, to eat right, to stop punishing the body with cigarettes, whiskey, and drugs, legal or illegal, to develop those good health habits, good mental habits, and good spiritual attitudes that lead to total fitness.

The Seven Deadly Sins include Pride, Covetousness, Lust, Anger, Envy, Gluttony, and Sloth. They are called deadly because fatal to spiritual progress. But "deadly" also means "likely to cause death; capable of causing death." Scientifically as well as spiritually, we know this at least is true of Gluttony and Sloth.

If there be some sacrifice in your new physical fitness approach to life, so be it. It's a small price to pay for the enormous benefits. When you begin to feel great again, when that wonderful feeling of health and vitality courses through your whole body as if reborn in a child, you'll wonder what took you so long.

Bibliography

Astrand, Per-Olof, *Health and Fitness*. Stockholm: Swedish Information Service, 1972.

Carlson, Duane R.; et al. (Editors), *Food & Fitness*. Chicago: The Blue Cross Association, 1973.

Cooper, Kenneth H., M.D., *The New Aerobics*. New York: M. Evans and Company, Inc., Bantam Books, 1970.

Cureton, Thomas K., Jr., *Physical Fitness and Dynamic Health*. New York: The Dial Press, 1965.

Friermood, Harold T. (Supervisor), *The YMCA Guide to Adult Fitness*. New York: Association Press, 1963.

Golding, L.; and Bos, R., *Scientific Foundations of Physical Fitness Programs*. Minneapolis, Minn.: Burgess Publishing Co., 1970.

Jokl, E., *Nutrition, Exercise, and Body Composition*. Springfield, Ill.: Charles C Thomas, Publisher, 1964.

Joseph, Jack J., "Physical Fitness Organization, Evaluation Program." (Unpublished manuscript.) Seattle, Wash.: YMCA, 1966.

Kasch, F. W.; and Boyer, J. L., *Adult Fitness, Principles and Practices*. Greeley, Colo.: All American Productions and Publications, 1968.

Kraus, H.; and Raab, W., *Hypokinetic Disease—Diseases Produced by Lack of Exercise*. Springfield, Ill.: Charles C Thomas, Publisher, 1961.

Kuntzleman, C., *The Physical Fitness Encyclopedia*. Emmaus, Pa. 18049: Rodale Books, Inc., 1970.

Kusinitz, Ivan; Freedman, Morris; and Fine, Morton, *The Challenge of Physical Fitness*. Westport, Conn.: Physical Fitness Laboratory Ltd., 1969.

Maness, Bill, *Exercise Your Heart*. London: The Macmillan Company, 1969.

Mayer, J., *Overweight: Causes, Cost and Control*. Englewood Cliffs, N.J.: Prentice-Hall, 1968.

Myers, Clayton R.; Golding, Lawrence A.; and Sinning, Wayne E. (Editors), *The Y's Way to Physical Fitness*. National Council YMCA, USA. Emmaus, Pa.: Rodale Press, 1973.

Myers, C. R., "Special Report, National YMCA Physical Fitness Consultation," *Journal of Physical Education,* March-April, 1972.

President's Council on Physical Fitness, The, *Adult Physical Fitness*. Washington, D.C.: U.S. Government Printing Office, 1963.

South Carolina Heart Association, "Proceedings of the National Workshop on Exercise in the Prevention, in the

Evaluation, in the Treatment of Heart Disease," *Journal of the South Carolina Medical Association.* Supplement to Vol. 65, No. 12, December, 1969. (Supplied by the South Carolina Heart Association, 2864 Devine Street, Columbia, S.C. 29205.)

Steinhaus, Arthur H., *How to Keep Fit and Like It.* Chicago: The Dartnell Corp., 1957.

Tennessee Heart Association Physical Exercise Committee, *Physician's Handbook for Evaluation of Cardiovascular and Physical Fitness.* Nashville, Tenn., 1972.

Williams, Richard L.; et al. (Editors), *The Healthy Life.* New York: Time-Life Books, 1966.

Index